ISBN: 978-0-9778874-7-7

For information about permission to reproduce selections from this book, write to Permissions, New Genius Media, 13681 Cedar Crest Lane 93K, Seal Beach, California 90740-4616. (310) 748-2409; (562) 598-9094

Or E-mail: Carl Bourhenne@gmail.com

Manufacturing by New Genius Media

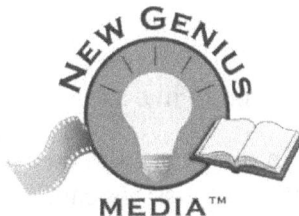

MEDIA™

<u>Nothing in this book is optional!</u>

If you eliminate something of this book from your lifestyle, replace it with something else that does the same thing, because everything in this book is necessary to live the longest life you possibly can.

If you want to live the longest life you can, you must follow **ALL** the precepts in this book.

I have spent the last 42 years researching how to live the longest life possible.

In 1976 I founded the Carl I. Bourhenne Medical Research Foundation to research the best ways to stay youthful, and to live the longest life possible.

I received Federal and State tax-exempt status for the Foundation, and it has been researching how to live the longest life possible ever since.

I went back to school in 1988 and earned a Master's Degree in Gerontology, the study of the aging process, from Cal State Dominguez.

In 2008 a member of a UCLA research group on anti-aging asked to be involved in my Foundation, and joined in. The Foundation is still active, and is still researching the ways to stay youthful and to live as long a life as is possible.

Follow my lead in this book, and do everything you can to live the longest life you possibly can.

The alternative is to die sooner than you should.

Carl Bourhenne, MA
Gerontologist

Carl Bourhenne's

FITNESS and LONG LIFE

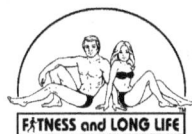

How To Live
The Longest Life Possible

Contents

No one should do anything affecting their lifestyle without first consulting their doctor.

3

FITNESS and LONG LIFE

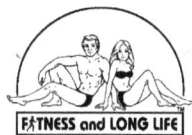

How To Live
The Longest Life Possible

Introduction

If you are not interested in living as long as you can, save yourself some time and stop reading here.

If you think you don't need to do anything to live as long as you can, or don't care how long you're going to live, don't bother reading any further.

The oldest **PROVEN** lifespan in the history of man was a woman named Jeanne Calment, who died in France in 1996 at the age of 121 years 164 days.

No one else in history has ever been proven to have lived that long, and every one of us is going to die well before the age of 120.

Research has shown that our human genes can support an absolute maximum of about 120 years of life. No one alive today will likely live that long.

How is your aging going? Feel less vigorous than you did a year ago? Less flexible? Have less energy…a LOT less? Moving a little slower? A LOT slower? Taking longer to think of names, or words? **I know how you feel! I used to feel like that.**

You are probably doing at least some of the things you know you must do to be healthy and to live the longest life that you possibly can; but it is also almost certain that you are **NOT** doing **ALL** the things that you must do to live the longest life that you can.

All of the changes that you are experiencing will get worse every day for the rest of your life, UNLESS YOU DO SOMETHING TO SLOW THEIR PROGRESS. You will get weaker in the knees and legs, and forget words and names more and more as time goes on.

Are you waiting for your youthfulness to return…to feel more like you felt yesterday? **YOUR HEALTH AND YOUTHFULNESS WILL NEVER RETURN UNLESS YOU IMPROVE YOUR LIFESTYLE IN CERTAIN NECESSARY WAYS!**

You CAN get back more strength in your legs and walk more strongly like you used to. You CAN get much of your youthfulness back, if you are willing to do the things that work, and if you don't wait too long! The longer you wait, the less you can get back!

My name is Carl Bourhenne, and 42 years ago I became aware that I am not going to live more than about 120 years. I became determined to live as long as I possibly can, and I've been investigating for the last 42 years how to live the longest life I possibly can.

I am 82 years old, I have no health problems, I take no medications, I run a mile and a half every day and lift weights four days, and I'm sexually active most days. I feel GREAT all the time! My blood pressure, cholesterol, and sugar are always normal.

I feel like I am 18 years old; but then I look in the mirror and realize that time marches on.

I have spent the last 42 years studying what we can do to fight the aging process, and to be youthful and live the longest life we possibly can. I will die one day, and you will too; but **I've learned all the ways to stay youthful and to live as long a life as we possibly can.**

It was in 1976 that I fully realized that I am going to get old and die before the age of 120, and that everyone else alive will too, including those that I love most.

So in 1976 I founded the Carl I. Bourhenne Medical Research Foundation to research the best ways to stay youthful, and to live the longest life possible. I received Federal and State tax-exempt status for the Foundation, and I've been researching long life ever since.

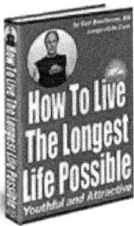

I went back to school in 1988 and earned a Master's Degree in Gerontology, the study of the aging process, from Cal State Dominguez.

My Master's Thesis was a work called, **"How To Live The Longest Life Possible."**

In 2008 a member of a UCLA research group on anti-aging asked to be involved in my Foundation, and joined in. The Foundation is still active, and is still researching the ways to stay youthful and to live as long a life as is possible.

I had always taken great care of myself until six years ago. Then I stopped living a healthy lifestyle for three years. **At the end of those three years, when I was 79, I was feeling a _lot_ of weakness in my legs, and I actually believed I'd need a walker very soon.**

I re-instated the lifestyle practices I had learned during my research, and I was surprised to find that **I returned to a vigorous youthfulness <u>very fast</u>! I promise to tell you ALL of the lifestyle practices that I used from my research.**

<u>**YOU CAN** maintain or regain much of your youthfulness, too</u>! There are definitely things that you can do to be more youthful and healthy, and to live the longest life you can. *But you must do them,* **or your aging and deterioration will continue, non-stop!**

<u>We all</u> have to do <u>all</u> of the things that I have learned, or we will all age continuously until our final day. **You can make the time between now and then completely different, if you are willing to do the things that work.** I promise to teach you **<u>all</u>** the things that actually work.

I will not try, in this short message, to list all of the important things that you **MUST** do to be youthful, and to live the longest life you possibly can. **Many people think they know it all, but <u>very few people</u> know <u>all the important things research shows that WE MUST DO</u>.**

Don't let another moment of your precious life and youthfulness slip away. **<u>If losses go on too long you can never get them back</u>!** I will show you **ALL** of the ways to live the longest life you can, healthy and youthful. **But _<u>YOU MUST DO THEM</u>_ or lose years of your life.**

    Carl Bourhenne, MA
    Gerontologist

Carl Bourhenne's

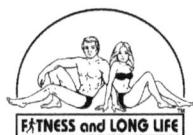

FITNESS and LONG LIFE

How To Live
The Longest Life Possible

Can You Live Forever?

(If not, how long **can** you live?)

"If I eat only healthy foods, if I exercise, if I never smoke or drink or use drugs, if I sleep right, if I get good medical care, if I control my weight, if I control stress, if I keep good social relations, if I keep a healthy mental attitude, if I never have an accident, if I stay excited about life - in short, if I inherited the best genes and take perfect care of myself,

Can I Live Forever?

And if not,

How Long **Can** I Live?

How long _is_ it possible for a human being to live? What is our **Maximum Potential Lifespan** (the longest a human being **can** live)? And, perhaps as important: can **we** influence the length, and the quality, of our lives?

Since every human being that has ever been born, unless dying prematurely has gotten old and died, the history of man shows us very clearly, that our life span so far has proven to be limited. This limit has been measured in terms that have generally been accepted by the communities of the gerontological, biological and anthropological sciences.

Richard G. Cutler at the Gerontology Research Center, Baltimore City Hospital, National Institute on Aging, National Institutes of Health has calculated the maximum life span for about 150 extinct mammalian species, and has also assessed the genetic potentials and traced the progress of the evolution of the Maximum Potential Lifespan of man.

The first truly human species was Homo habilis which emerged from Australopithecus africanus about 1.8 million years ago. Homo Sapiens evolved about 100,000 years ago. The Maximum Potential Life Span of our species was increasing at a very fast rate until about 100,000 years ago when the increase suddenly stopped, and has since remained fixed at about 120 years.

What Is The Longest Known Lifespan?

The oldest **PROVEN** lifespan in the history of man was a woman named Jeanne Calment, who died in France in 1996 at the age of 121 years 164 days.

No one else in history has ever been proven to have lived that long, and every one of us is going to die well before the age of 120.

Research has shown that our human genes can support an absolute maximum of about 120 years of life. No one alive today will likely live that long.

You have undoubtedly read about claims of unusually long life by various individuals and societies, such as the three areas of the world where claims of unusually

long life abound.
1. **The Abkhasians in the Caucasus Mountains of Soviet Georgia.** (The most famous)
2. **The Vilcabambans in the Ecuadorian Andes.**
2. **The Hunzas in the Karakorum Mountains of Kashmir in West Pakistan's Himalayas.**

The claims of 150 plus years among the Abkhasians have all been proven false though, by two men named Zhores Medvedev, a leading Russian investigator of aging, and Alexander Leaf of the Harvard Medical School. These two researchers investigated, and they found falsification of birth dates and ages for such reasons as the avoidance of military service, and the promotion of tourism. **They had adopted their father's identities.**

It is interesting to note, though, that these three areas all have an unusually large number of people over the age of 100, and they all are also hilly country where the people walk instead of ride. They also all have diets high in vegetables and grains, and low in meats.

As of the completion of this writing, **the longest proven life span in the history of mankind is that of Jeanne Louise Calment.** She was born in France on February 21, 1875 and died in August 1997 at the age of **121 years six months.** As of this writing, the longest-lived person in the United Stated was Carrie White, who was born on November 18, 1874 and died on February 14, 1991 at the age of 116 years, 88 days.

Maximum Potential Lifespan Vs. Life Expectancy

Besides the idea of our **Maximum Potential Lifespan** (the longest anyone **can** live) of about 120 years, we also talk about your own **Life Expectancy** = how long you will **probably live** within your 120 year maximum potential.

Can we control our own Life Expectancy -- how long we will probably live, within our 120-year Maximum Potential Lifespan?

The medical and biological sciences have shown that we can control, to a significant degree, not only the length but also the quality of our life. Although we cannot at present extend our Maximum Potential Lifespan of about 120 years, we can influence how many of our 120 years we do live. And research is going on around the world to try to learn how to extend our lives beyond 120 years - healthy, attractive, and youthful.

At present, **Genetic Engineering** appears to hold the best answer, especially after we complete a "map" of where each of the genes are on each of our chromosomes **Mapping the Human Genome)**.

The average life expectancy of the cave man was about 16 years. In 500 BC the average life expectancy was about 20 years. In 400 AD it was 35 years. In 1900 it was 47 years. In 1930 it was 59 years. By 1975 it had advanced to about 71 years, and in 1989 it had advanced to 74 years for men and 78 years for women. Speculatively, by the year 2,010 it might be 100 years. During all of these times the Maximum Potential Lifespan remained at about 120 years, and has not increased.

The major differences in lifestyle and the hardship factors alone make the reasons for the difference in life expectancy during the nineteenth century pretty obvious. Pre-natal care, post-natal care, better quality child protection and care, much easier and less exposed living conditions, better nutrition, and better medical care account for much of the difference in life expectancy between then and now.

The extraordinary increase in average life expectancy in the U.S. during the nineteenth century though, is due mainly to advances in sanitation, public health, and medicine. At all

12

age levels, prevention and cure have played a major part. The adoption of sterilization techniques by doctors drastically reduced the deaths of women in childbirth. Treatment for some childhood diseases such as measles, polio, chicken pox, whooping cough, and bacterial infections helped to sharply reduce the deaths of infants and children. Tuberculosis has been virtually eradicated. Medical science has truly advanced dramatically during the nineteenth century. It has been said that if a medical doctor fell asleep in the year 1900 and woke up in 1930, he would still have been able to practice medicine. But if a doctor fell asleep in 1930 and awoke in 1960, he would have had about the same knowledge as a first year medical student.

The medical and health literature is filled with research results and instructions for optimizing our lifespan and the quality of that life, by following healthy lifestyle habits. The American Heart Association, The American Lung Association, The American Cancer Society, and many other such quality organizations regularly distribute information describing research-based methods for protecting our health, and optimizing our life expectancy. Based on this and other information, insurance companies gamble billions of dollars per year that they can accurately predict the length of your life, and they win.

They base their life insurance programs on factors of heredity, and of lifestyle. Cuna Mutual Insurance Group of Madison, Wisconsin circulated an At-Home Longevity Test, as a part of a sales packet. In order to determine your own life expectancy, it provided a questionnaire, and 24 of the 29 questions relate to lifestyle, with 5 relating to heredity. So lifestyle practices are well established as major determinants of how long we can expect to live within our 120 year maximum, and also of the quality of that life.

A nd this book, **How To Live The Longest Life Possible**, is designed to help you to live to your Maximum Potential Lifespan, healthy, attractive, and youthful. One of the reasons this book is needed is because of the low quality and so often erroneous information with which we are constantly bombarded.

For example, in a wide variety of media recently, we read and heard that we must ingest large amounts of Calcium in order to prevent bone loss (osteoporosis) as we age, especially for women. So, many people are ingesting large amounts of Calcium supplements. Is this healthy? Perhaps not. The New England Journal of Medicine provides very important research-based information, but it will reach relatively few eyes and ears: The <u>form</u> of Calcium supplementation is important. Calcium carbonate causes kidney stones, and calcium gluconate tablets are too large to swallow comfortably for many people. Calcium citrate might be the best form of calcium supplement. And although ingestion of adequate amounts of Calcium is necessary for normal bone-forming activities, larger doses will not slow bone loss. Excess Calcium ingestion causes calcification of the heart valves, and kidney stones. So, about 800 mg. per day of calcium citrate (about 1500 mg. per day for women after menopause) appears to be the best form. Of course, **only your doctor can determine the best amount and form for you**.

Also, moderate stress on the bones (such as during exercise) has been shown to deter bone loss by stimulating the action of bone forming cells called osteoblasts. For this reason, swimming does little to fight osteoporosis because it places little stress on the bones. Walking, jogging, and weight training do more to prevent osteoporosis.

Also, some simple facts are not commonly known, such as the fact known in geriatric medicine but not widely disseminated, that straining at the stool in earlier years

14

(pushing too hard while on the toilet) can cause many cases of diverticular disease, hemorrhoids, and incontinence later in life.

Also important is the fact that many popular myths need to be exposed, dispelling the sometimes terrifying fears which arise from some of the myths. Perhaps the most significant factors regarding the lack of information and the bad information that are common, are the detriments to health and longevity that are accruing at this moment to those lacking accurate information.

Carl Bourhenne, MA
Gerontologist

FITNESS and LONG LIFE

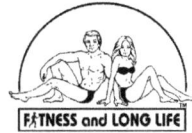

How To Live
The Longest Life Possible

Why We Age

The Five Major Theories

Why don't we just "live forever"? Why do some people die sooner than others? What can we do to stay healthy and youthful, and live longer? What new technologies are being developed? Will man someday be able to live forever, except for major accidents? These are the questions that originally stimulated my interest.

What does cause death, and why don't we just "live forever"?

About 100 years ago Mathias Schwann and Theodore Schweiden recognized that the cell is the fundamental unit of all living organisms.
Millions of cells make up our skin and our muscles. No matter what living organism we examine, we will always find that it is composed of cells. When cells get worn out, most of them divide and form new cells (post-fixed mitotic cells, such as nerve cells cannot). All of the basic biochemical processes take place or begin in the cell.

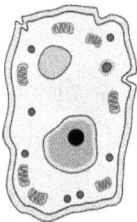

In youth during our growth period (up to about 18 years of age), the number of newly formed cells in our body outnumbers dying cells. In young adulthood, from about 18 to about 25 years of age, the number of newly formed cells balances the dying cells. In aging (after 25 years of age) the number of newly formed cells is less than the number of cells that die.

Aging is cells dying faster than they are replaced, or losing some of their functioning.

In 1961 Dr. Leonard Hayflick at Stanford University discovered that human cells growing in a culture of energy and nutrients could reproduce themselves only a limited number of times before all of their descendants aged and died. The maximum number of times a cell can reproduce itself is now called its "Hayflick limit".

Each type of cell has its own Hayflick limit. Dr. Hayflick also showed that long before cells ceased to reproduce themselves they showed certain changes in their structure and functioning, such as less ability to produce energy, less ability to make enzymes quickly enough, and more waste materials inside each cell.

So Dr. Hayflick concluded that these age changes in the cells play the central role in the expression of aging in the body, and result in the death of the individual well before all of its cells fail to divide.

Death is caused by the loss of too many cells, or the loss of cell function. Many theories have been proposed to explain how Hayflick's limit is expressed in the cells in our bodies. All of them assume that aging represents a loss of control over various bodily processes, and many of them assume that the loss of control occurs at the cellular level in the DNA of those cells.

The Five Major Theories Of Why We Age

1. The Error Hypothesis
2. The Free Radical Theory
3. The Cross-linkage Theory
4. The Brain Hypothesis
5. The Autoimmune Theory

1. The Error Hypothesis:

The Error Hypothesis, or "aging by mistake", refers to the errors which may occur in the chemical reactions in producing DNA, RNA, or proteins, because the metabolic machinery is not 100% accurate. Cell death can result from these unrepaired errors. Some gerontologists attribute this error to any one, or a combination of the following: Insufficient energy or nutrients, or insufficient carrying away of cell waste products.

2. The Free Radical Theory:

The Free Radical Theory refers to molecules, which have a strong tendency to link to other molecules, interfering with their functioning. They are produced by cells to assist in metabolism, most commonly in the "burning" of sugar. They are sometimes produced by accident if oxygen, always present in the cell and highly reactive, combines with cellular molecules. Uncontrolled free radicals can cause accumulated damage to the membranes surrounding cells and to the cellular molecules of DNA and RNA. Sufficient damage results in the eventual death of the cell.

At present the Free Radical theory is being hotly investigated. Research on mice shows that a 40% reduction in calorie intake results in a doubling of their life span. When food is metabolized, free radicals are produced. Our bodies do produce free radical "sponges" which absorb free radicals, but often not enough. The ingestion of vitamins E and C are especially good free radical absorbers.

3. The Cross-linkage Theory:

The Cross-linkage Theory states that the aging of living organisms is due to the occasional formation, by cross-linkage, of bridges between protein molecules in the DNA which cannot be broken by the cell repair enzymes, interfering in the production of RNA by DNA. Cross-linkages in protein and DNA can be caused by many chemicals normally present in cells as a result of metabolism, and by common pollutants such as lead and tobacco smoke.

4. The Brain Hypothesis:

The Brain Hypothesis, or breakdown of the brain pacemaker, refers to the theory that aging is due to a breakdown in the homeostasis of the bodily functions - especially in the control of the hypothalamus over the pituitary - which in turn causes a breakdown in control over the endocrine glands.

5. The Autoimmune Theory:

The Autoimmune Theory, proposed by Dr. Roy Walford at UCLA hypothesizes that two types of white blood cells, B and T cells of the immune system weaken with age, and malfunction. B cells lose their vigor in attacking bacteria, viruses, and cancer cells, and the T cells lose their vigor in attacking cells foreign to the body, such as cancer cells and transplant cells. When B and T cells malfunction, they attack normal healthy body cells.

Carl Bourhenne, MA
Gerontologist

Carl Bourhenne's

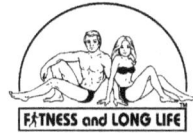

FITNESS and LONG LIFE

How To Live
The Longest Life Possible

How Our Body Changes As We Age
Each Body Part

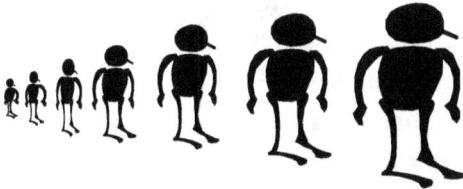

It is no secret that as we age our bodies change, and that the changes in mid-life and middle age tend to be deleterious to our health. Research has also clearly shown that our lifestyle impacts both positively and negatively on these changes. The need to attend to our health by attending to our lifestyle is subscribed to by such revered organizations as the aforementioned American Heart Association, The American Cancer Society, The American Lung Association, and the many other highly regarded health-related organizations with which we are all familiar. We are advised to pay great attention to what we eat, to exercise regularly, not to perform such harmful activities as smoking or using recreational drugs, and so to preserve our physical and mental capabilities.

How Do Our Bodies Change With Age?

What are the changes, and the sequence of the changes that our bodies undergo as we age, and what effect do these changes have on our health status? What are the social implications? Perhaps most important, what are the alternatives?

In order to summarize the many ways our bodies change with age, I have organized the changes according to our body systems.

The Body Systems:
1. The Skin
2. The Skeletal System
3. The Muscular System
4. The Neurosensory System
5. The Gastrointestinal Tract
6. The Cardiopulmonary System
7. The Cerebrovascular System
8. The Urinary System
9. The Endocrine System
10. The Genital System
11. The Immune System

The reasons for, and the details of the physiological processes of these changes are not within the purview or the space allowance of this book, so I will merely state the changes, and address the subsequent issues in their regard.

The reader will please be aware that, not only do people "age" at radically different rates of change, but also within each person, the various parts and systems "age" at different - often radically different - rates.

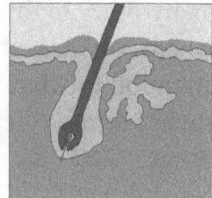

1. The Skin:

As the skin ages, it flattens due to the loss of: sub-cutaneous fat, skin cells, sebaceous (oil) glands, sweat glands, melanocytes (pigment cells), and hair follicles. Lentigo (senile freckles) occur, blood flow to the skin is decreased, and nerve endings are lost or become less sensitive.

As a result, the skin loses some of its effectiveness: as a protector against bacteria, as an insulator, as a thermal regulator, and as a sensory receptor. Since these losses cause wrinkling, loss of elasticity, freedom of movement and expression are inhibited. The slowing of circulation results in slower healing. The loss of color is also seen, as the hair becomes gray.

The skin generally functions well throughout life though, and most changes in the skin due to aging are not life-threatening. Most of the deleterious changes in the skin are cosmetic, as the drying and thinning result in sagging and wrinkling, the hair becomes sparser and gray or white, and the fingernails become ridged, tend to yellow, and are prone to splitting.

Skin disorders more common in the aging skin are senile pruritis (itching), keratoses (thickening in patches), skin cancer, and decubitus ulcers (pressure sores), and herpes zoster (shingles).

The social implications of these effects are based, in the United States, on a significant cultural tendency toward ageism in virtually all of its forms. One's social life becomes more limited as younger people view elders as "not fun", "slow", "grumpy", and so on. These views spill into the work-place or what might be a potential work-place, as one who looks "old" is not considered as having much to offer.

The alternatives involve personal effort by the elders in making as much of an effort as they are capable in relating to others, social responsibility by the community to understand the limitations of the elderly and provide a social environment based on actual conditions rather than assumed limitations.

The elderly themselves have a direction for alternatives, biologically, to varying degrees. They can avoid excessive exposure to the sun, maintain moisture in the skin, provide adequate nutrition so that the skin can be maintained and repaired, and get regular exercise to maintain circulation in the skin.

2. The Skeletal System:

The primary factor in the aging of the skeletal system is the loss of bone matter. This loss is called osteoporosis, and refers to bone loss. The basic cause of bone loss is the fact that the relative rates of production of osteoblasts (bone forming cells) and osteoclasts (bone dissolving cells) changes so that more bone matter is dissolved than is laid down. This loss is much greater in women than in men.

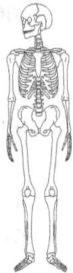

Other factors in the aging skeletal system are loosened cartilage around the joints, depleted lubricating fluid in the joints, and hardened and contracted ligaments. These factors occur more in men than in women.

The effects of these changes on our health status are significant. Bones become brittle and less supportive of our activities, resulting in less activity, which in turn results in poorer health. The excess bone taken up tends to reside in the arteries and local blood vessels, causing decreased circulation. As broken bones occur, less mobilization results in other health hazards.

The social implications of these effects are widespread, especially in advanced conditions. One becomes more dependent upon others, who might begin to avoid. One is less able to visit and to participate in social events.

The alternatives to immobilization are difficult. Family, friends, and the community must be open to assisting these individuals, and must be alert to avoid ascribing more limitations than are actual. Other alternatives are preventive techniques.

The following diseases tend to increase the incidence of osteoporosis, and so should be treated diligently: chronic alcoholism, diabetes, hyperthyroidism, uremia, and collagen disease (rheumatoid arthritis).

The current fad of ingesting large quantities of calcium in the diet can be dangerous, and have not been shown to significantly control osteoporosis. In fact, excess calcium ingestion causes calcification of the heart valves.

The most successful deterrent to osteoporosis so far has been the stress placed upon the bones by exercise, which appears to stimulate the activity of osteoblasts (bone forming cells).

3. The Muscular System:

Since muscle cells are postmitotic cells (unable to replace themselves once they are formed), all muscle cell loss is permanent. Even though muscular response gradually slows with age even under the best conditions, the loss of muscular capabilities is by far mostly the result of cell loss due to **inactivity**. As muscle cells are lost, weakness and slowness increase.

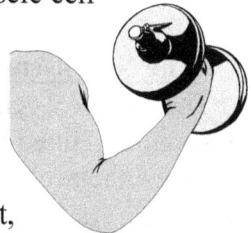

The effects of these changes on our health status are not, in themselves, greatly deleterious. The muscles, however, are the main tools for effecting strong circulation throughout the body.

The social implications of these changes are related both to appearance and to movement.

As the muscles become smaller, including the muscles in the face, and as adipose (fat) tissue accumulates, including in the face, the entire appearance changes to that of an older person, with all the ramifications described above in the description of skin changes. In addition, as muscle fibers decrease, weaken, and slow, it becomes increasingly difficult to keep up with younger people, who may make allowances, but who may also become avoidant.

The alternatives to these conditions can be social allowances and patience, which are sometimes offered; but, social programs such as the Senior Olympics not only help keep seniors healthier and more active, but also more capable of keeping up with younger people and of relating to them better.

The left ventricle of the heart, and the diaphragm do not lose muscle fibers with age, because they are continually active. A well designed, consistently followed exercise program is indispensable for the maintenance of muscle cells, and of good health over time.

4. **The Neurosensory System**:
The nerve cells (neurons) are postmitotic fixed cells (unable to replace themselves once they are formed). As they age, they lose dendrites, dendritic spines, and end branches; all of which are the intermediary parts necessary for the communication with one another. As the nervous system ages, signal conduction slows, but much more so at the nerve

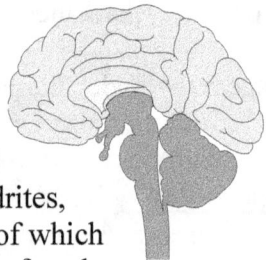

26

synapses (nerve junctions) than within the nerve cells themselves. We lose taste buds, olfactory cells (sense of smell), nerve endings in the skin, and even brain cells. Our hearing loses sensitivity, especially in the higher ranges, as the ear ossicles harden. Our vision changes as the lens of the eye becomes less flexible and yellows, and we require more light and glasses for close work.

The effects of these changes on our health status impact on the ability to drive, read, and communicate; but the most relevant loss is a lessening of ability to organize and integrate information as well. The subsequent lessening of ability to care for oneself can impact on health in many ways.

The social implications of these changes are especially significant as communications slow and others become impatient with the slowness and memory deficits, which sometimes occur. Others may avoid the elderly, become impatient with them, and the elderly may then become less interested in interacting.

The alternatives are greater social awareness and allowance. It is also important for the elderly to be as mentally active as possible, in order to alleviate the effects of slowing as much as possible. In fact, a mind kept well active need not lose any significant functioning, including memory; and a re-activated mind may regain most or all of its normal functioning, if it is not diseased.

5. The Gastrointestinal Tract:

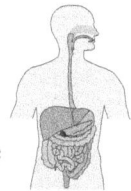

The mouth, esophagus, stomach, small intestine, gallbladder, liver, pancreas, and large intestine compose the Gastrointestinal tract.

In the mouth, taste buds and teeth are lost. Problems with the esophagus in aging can be dysphagia (difficulty swallowing), substernal pain, heartburn, belching, and general epigastric discomfort. Atrophic changes in the stomach, especially hypoacidity and achlorhydria, are common as we age. Cell replacement is active in the small intestine, so few changes occur with aging; but obstructions are not uncommon.

Gallbladder problems are most marked after age 65, rather than in middle age. Also, the body's largest gland, the liver, maintains most of its weight until about age 70, and for the non-alcoholic can remain quite healthy and normal. Problems with the pancreas usually begin to develop about age 40 if they do occur, but they do tend to increase with age, especially if the Islets of Langerhans are damaged, or if they become over stressed by excess sugar consumption. In those instances, diabetes develops.

The large intestine is most susceptible to disease with aging, but is also most amenable to preventive measures. Obstructions of the bowel - carcinogenic or otherwise, diverticular disease, hemorrhoids, and Gastrointestinal discomfort are common in the elderly, as is fecal incontinence. These latter problems can cause a severe strain on one's self-image, but many can often be avoided by simply avoiding straining at the stool early in life.

The effects of these changes on our health status can be far-reaching, because they can affect our nutritional sustenance. Every aspect of our health is endangered by severe problems in the gastrointestinal tract.

The social implications of these effects relate mainly to the results of most illnesses, except for fecal incontinence, with its obvious discomforts and embarrassments, but which is often easily prevented by not straining at the stool early in life. Straining at the stool weakens the sphincter muscle over time.

The alternatives to the problems of these illnesses are, again, some re-education and change of attitudes in the community. The alternatives from a biological perspective are, as mentioned, preventive; with the greatest opportunities for prevention being in the regular consumption of fiber.

6. The Cardiopulmonary System:

Heart disease is the most common cause of death in people 65 and over, and is also the most frequent cause of activity limitations. The heart muscles reduce in size and the aorta loses some of its elasticity. Coronary artery disease increases as activity declines. Plaques accumulate on the interior of the arteries (atherosclerosis), and the arteries harden as they lose their elasticity (arteriosclerosis); both of these factors resulting in lessened blood flow.

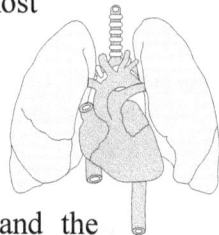

Hypertension (high blood pressure) also increases with age. Several factors can stimulate the onset of congestive heart failure, and all are related to excessive demand on the right side of the heart.

The respiratory system also undergoes changes with age. The air sacs, airways, and tissues lose elasticity and become more rigid. In general however, serious disease notwithstanding, the respiratory system can serve one well throughout life. The effects of these changes on our health status need not be severe without such abuses as smoking.

The social implications of the effects of these changes are often not such as would hamper reasonable normal functioning.

The alternatives are not socially demanding, and the biological changes can be greatly diminished by a regular, strenuous exercise regimen that causes deep breathing over a period of time.

7. The Cerebrovascular System:

Atherosclerosis (plaque formation inside the arteries) and arteriosclerosis (hardening of the arteries) in the blood vessels that supply the brain is called cerebrovascular disease, and causes strokes. Prior to the complete occlusion of the blood vessels, the brain is deprived of adequate blood flow resulting in less than optimal brain functioning, such as confusion, disorientation, and memory loss. Strokes may result in hemiplegia (paralysis), aphasia (speech disorder), and sensory deprivation in varying degrees.

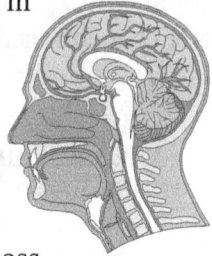

The effects of these changes on our health status can be drastic, ranging from slight discomfort to death.

The social implications of these effects can also be severe, as those suffering these indignities become less functional both mentally and physically; and are, in varying degrees a burden to others. Social interactions are doubly inhibited, as from inside, the patient is less able to interact; and from outside, family, friends, and others may be less interested in interacting.

The alternatives are an enhancement of understanding by the community and, before the fact, preventive measures such as diet and exercise, which have been shown to decrease or even prevent cerebrovascular accidents.

8. The Urinary System:

The bladder, urethra, urinary tract, prostate, and kidneys all show decremental incidence in most people with age. Urinary incontinence and urinary tract infections are the most common problems encountered. The capacity of the bladder reduces by half in the elderly, so there is a need to urinate more frequently.

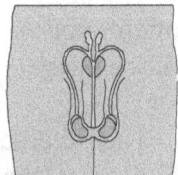

From the age of 50 on prostate problems increase in frequency in men. A decrease in the number of nephrons, the filtering module of the kidney, results in decrease efficiency of the kidneys.

The effects of these changes on our health status range from mild to severe. While 50% of the elderly have no significant urinary health problems, less than 4% have no deterioration.

The social implications of these effects can be mild, or severe if there is great incontinence or severe kidney failure.

The alternatives must include great compassion and understanding in either case, but the best course of action is good health practices throughout life to maintain the urinary system in good health.

9. The Endocrine System:

To some researchers the endocrine system is the most exciting area of research into the basic cause of aging.   The pituitary, thyroid, and adrenal glands do, however, tend   to function adequately throughout life. While size of the thyroid gland does decrease significantly with age, it is the young and middle aged who experience thyroid problems rather than the elderly.

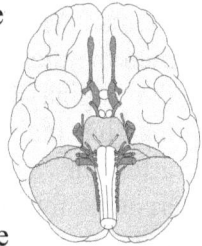

The effects of these changes on our health status can by significant, especially in the event of diabetes; otherwise however, the endocrine system serves us well in our old age.

The social implications of these effects are not a major cause for concern for most people. Diabetics require special consideration in severe instances, but for most caregivers and social interactions this is not a large problem.

The alternatives to be dealt with are primarily the self-care factors for avoiding the onset of diabetes. It is prevalent with urbanization, civilized work patterns, sedentary lifestyles, and a modern diet.

10. The Genital System:

The changes in the genital system tend to be non-problematic, especially if sexuality has been practiced without long periods of abstinence. The changes that do occur are not as age related as they are sexuality related. Generally, responses slow gradually in both men and women, but both can have normal sexual relations as long as they are healthy, at any age. The subject of optimal sexuality is not an issue of this book, and is not truly an issue of aging. It is more an issue of education and psychological response, since the body changes are not age significant.

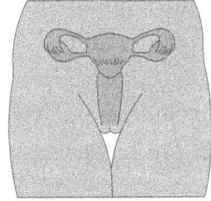

In men, the prostate may enlarge, and may create urinary problems. More changes occur in women than in men. In women the uterus atrophies some, and several changes occur in the vagina; but all can be dealt with, especially if the woman has maintained some regular level of sexual activity. If after the age of about 40 a woman abstains from intercourse for prolonged periods, 3 to 5 years, the ability to secrete lubricating fluids, and much of the elasticity of the vagina are permanently lost. Masturbation can effectively help to maintain both of these capabilities, especially if object insertion is included. Since most research shows that less than 50% of women practice object insertion during masturbation, these women who also abstain from intercourse lose some vaginal elasticity, even with regular masturbation.

The effects of these changes on our health status are not significant, given the above conditions. In the case of prostate problems in men, difficulties can occur.

The social implications of these effects need not be severely problematic in most cases, remembering that most sexual problems are social or psychological problems which occur at all ages.

In the event that the woman has been sexually abstinent for a period of 3 to 5 years or more, the use of K-Y Jelly or some other **non-alcoholic, non-petroleum** lubricant designed for compatibility with the chemistry of the vagina may adequately alleviate discomfort in sexual intercourse. **Petroleum products such as baby oil and vaseline must never be put in or on the vagina, as they will upset the pH balance of the vagina, making it susceptible to yeast infections and other problems.**

The alternatives to these effects are activity, especially continued regular sexual activity, exercise, good nutrition, and good health habits.

11. The Immune System:

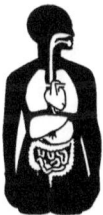

The earliest deterioration in our bodies is seen in the thymus - the heart of the immune system. The thymus begins significant involution in all of us by the age of three years. Two types of white blood cells, B cells and T cells of the immune system malfunction and weaken with age. B cells lose their vigor in attacking bacteria, viruses, and cancer cells; and the T cells lose their vigor in attacking cells foreign to the body, such as cancer cells and transplant cells. B cells and T cells also malfunction and attack normal healthy body cells.

Since our immune system is strongly impacted by our emotions and our moods, less enthusiasm for life or depression over reduced vigor or lost relationships can promote a circle of lessening health.

The old saying, **"Use it, or lose it"** is evermore confirmed by the ongoing research which continues to show that age-related losses in body functioning, and thus in health and long life, are very often a result of disuse, or of a lack of oxygen, nutrients, or body chemicals due to an insufficiency of circulation of the blood throughout the body, as a result of inactivity. If we use, and so maintain our functions, many of the problems related to aging would be experienced for a much shorter period of time, and many not at all.

Carl Bourhenne, MA
   Gerontologist

Carl Bourhenne's

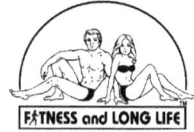

FITNESS and LONG LIFE

How To Live
The Longest Life Possible

How To Live The Longest Life Possible

I began to notice my father starting to show his age. That was when I began to do research on the human aging process, with the idea of learning all of the ways to deter aging, and discover or formulate new ways.

During these past thirty-two years I have earned a Master's Degree in Gerontology (the study of the aging process) from California State University, and in 1976 I founded a California non-profit corporation to perform research on the aging process. After one name change, **it is now called The Carl I. Bourhenne Medical Research Foundation.** Shortly after it was founded, it was granted Federal and State tax exempt status.

I returned to school in 1988 and earned a Master's Degree in Gerontology, the study of the aging process. My Master's Thesis was a work entitles, HOW TO LIVE THE LONGEST LIFE POSSIBLE

My studies and research have yielded many, many ways in which we can influence our own individual aging and help us to live the longest life possible, youthful and attractive.

I have organized these lifestyle practices and information into thireen categories, and my research and studies of the past (and continuing) twenty-four years is contained herein.

The Thirteen lifestyle practices <u>THAT WE HAVE CONTROL OF</u> that we must practice to stay healthy and Live The Longest Life Possible are:

Exercise

Nutrition

Sleep

Medical Care

Stress Control

Weight Management

Stay Active

Social Activity

Smoking, Drinking, Drugs

Safety

Environmental Concerns

Financial Security (Read this section well!)

Psychological: What you <u>like</u> to do, Expectations

Carl Bourhenne, MA
Gerontologist

Carl Bourhenne's

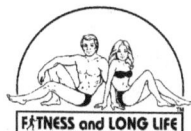

FITNESS and LONG LIFE

How To Live
The Longest Life Possible

Exercise

If you were to ask for a **Miracle Pill** that would likely prevent diabetes, heart problems, high blood pressure, high cholesterol, dementia, stiffness of the joints, and muscle weakness, you would find one.

There is such a "Pill", and it is not only inexpensive but it's actually free. **It's called, EXERCISE,** because it can do all those things in most people, if they do it regularly and diligently.

So, <u>THERE IS NO ALTERNATIVE TO EXERCISE</u> to maintain youthfulness and long life. The huge army of researchers around the world are experimenting with methods, ingestions, and substances. **<u>Nothing else does what only exercise accomplishes.</u>**

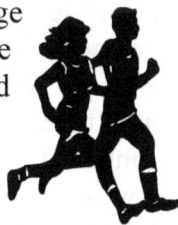

Along with calorie reduction, exercise can be one of the most influential factors on your longevity, health, attractiveness, and youthfulness. And it is easy to understand why the successful professional athlete follows a well designed program of physical fitness on a consistent basis. And yet, we all share the same basic anatomy and physiology, and thus the same essential need for physical fitness.

The three components of physical fitness are the same for all of us:

Strength, Flexibility, and Stamina.

Strength is developed and maintained by overcoming resistance. The best forms of strength development and maintenance are weight training, push-ups, pull-ups, sit-ups, and calisthenics. The broader the range of movement and angles of application, the more effective the strength development.

Flexibility refers to the capability of muscles, ligaments, tendons, and bones to provide a wide range of movement in joints. Muscles, ligaments, tendons, and bones all have a degree of elasticity which varies according to the degree and frequency to which the elasticity is practiced. Flexibility is developed and maintained by regular, gentle stretching routines.

Stamina, or endurance, refers to the ability to sustain activity for a period of time. Stamina, as with most other human abilities, comes from practice - that is performing full-body activities involving the large muscles and major joints for a period of time. Stamina can be developed and maintained by walking, running, bicycling, swimming, and by weight training with lighter weights and many repetitions. The main way that stamina develops is by increasing the ability of the body - especially the muscles - to transport oxygen. Stamina training results in the formation of a larger number of capillaries throughout the muscles, and is also the training necessary for cardio-vascular health.

In order for Strength, Flexibility, and Stamina to be developed and maintained, exercise sessions must be both frequent and reasonably intense. Naturally, intensity must be relatively low in the beginning, and should be increased as conditioning is developed.

The benefits of a regular exercise program are so profound as to affect the entire person physically, mentally, emotionally, socially, and vocationally. Many people say they actually feel like a different person. This is not surprising, in view of the fact that exercise causes the brain to produce "**endorphins**", a natural substance with the same general chemistry as morphine. It makes us feel good and accounts for the feeling of "runner's high" that many distance runners experience. It would be hard to argue against the statement that "exercise makes happiness".

The exercised person is leaner, stronger, has better circulation, recovers more quickly after exercise, illness, and other life changes; and is better protected against illness, especially cardio-vascular disease.

Some evidence shows that there is a relationship between regular exercise and physiological aging. The unexercised person often displays physical characteristics of early aging, with physiological middle-age arriving before the chronological age middle age. On the other hand, exercised individuals in their 60's and older can be vigorous "youngsters".

Indeed, research shows that regular exercise postpones physiological aging in adulthood, and enhances strength and stamina in old age. Problematic, though, is the fact that declining suppleness results from the accumulation of major and minor injuries of the joints. Since joint damage and deterioration are not presently reversible great care must be taken throughout life to avoid injury or undue stress to the joints.

Following is a list of research-documented physiological effects of regular, strenuous exercise:

Decreased body fat, increased lean body weight (muscles, etc.), increased strength/weight ratio, lower resting heart rate, more ATP (the energy currency in muscles), faster return of heart rate and blood pressure to normal after exercise, improved stroke volume of the heart, lowered blood lactates (fatigue products) for given work load, lowered heart rate during moderate work, increased lung capacity (Vital Capacity, and Tidal Air), increased maximum oxygen debt - blood lactates at maximal work, increased oxygen extraction at tissues during maximal work, increased aerobic capacity of maximal oxygen uptake per body weight or body surface area, lowered blood lipids (cholesterol, triglycerides, etc.), increased HDL (high density lipoprotein - the good one), increased blood volume and total hemoglobin (overall oxygen-carrying capacity), increased bone density and joint strength, increased cardiac and skeletal muscle vascularization, increased digestive efficiency and bowel functions, less postural problems and low back pain, less emotional disturbances (esp. anxiety and depression); and, decreased chronic fatigue, shortness of breath, overweight, digestive upsets, headache, backache, anxiety states, muscular weakness and atrophy, musculosketal (muscle, bone, joint, ligament, tendon) pain and injuries, high blood pressure, atherosclerosis, coronary artery disease, and generalized, accelerated degenerative aging.

It is interesting to note that exercise is presently the best known way to prevent osteoporosis if the exercise places stress on the bones. Calcium ingestion simply hardens the existing bone tissue, but stress on the bones (such as from most types of exercise) stimulates the production of bone forming cells (osteoblasts), deterring osteoporosis.

As great as any of the other benefits of exercise is the fact that it generates a release of the tension caused by stress.

This tension is represented by restricted arterioles, high blood pressure, and increased heart rate.

For those who still wonder if strenuous exercise is dangerous as we age, observe the results of a study of more than one million men and women over a six year period:

Death per 100 persons from coronary heart disease by degree of exertion:

Age	No Exercise	Slight Exercise	Moderate Exercise	Heavy Exercise
40-49	1.46	1.17	1.12	1.00
50-59	1.43	1.17	1.06	1.00
60-69	1.91	1.64	1.19	1.00
70-79	2.91	2.03	1.45	1.00

The conclusion is obvious: The more strenuous the exercise, the lower the death rate in each age group.

Exercises for the promotion of a healthy cardiovascular system are the same as those which promote stamina.

Some precautions should be noted in doing cardio-vascular exercises, especially running:
1. Warm up for 2 to 10 minutes. Do not stretch cold muscles, tendons, and ligaments, as they are stiff and will tear. Stretch only after an adequate warm-up.
2. Start slowly and progress gradually.
3. Exercise before eating, or wait 2 hours after eating.
4. Exercise in temperatures between 40ø and 85ø F, with humidity under 60%. Do not wear rubber or plastic suits.
5. Avoid standing still immediately after exercising. Cool down by slow walking or similar means for 10 minutes before a hot shower.
6. When not feeling up to par and after illness do not exercise, or exercise at a lower level. One of the important reasons to begin an exercise program at a slow

pace and build up over time is for the joints. When they do not have elasticity they are subject to **irreversible** injury. Also, when the thigh muscles are weak, the knees are subject to irreversible injury. Reasonable, but not severe musculoskeletal pains are common during the first two weeks, but should disappear shortly thereafter.

7. Do not drink alcoholic beverages for at least two hours prior to exercising.

8. Do not sprint at the end of your work-out.

9. If you experience any of the following during or after exercising, discontinue your exercise and consult your doctor: Pain in the chest, teeth, jaw, neck, or arm; significant difficulty in breathing; Light-headedness or fainting; Irregular heart rate, persisting during exercise and recovery period; Disabling musculoskeletal discomfort or swelling of joints; Excess fatigue as indicated by constant lethargy, malaise (indefinite discomfort), or an uncoordinated gate with weakness after exercise; Unexplained notable weight loss; Persistent nausea or vomiting after exercise.

A**void overexertion**, since it both predisposes to injury, and does not contribute to overall fitness. Steady progress is the fastest way to peak conditioning.

The Following Are Signs Of Overexertion:

Pulse rate not recovered to 120 beats per minute or lower within two minutes of stopping exercise. Feelings of fatigue persisting more than 10 minutes after end of work-out. Persistent difficulty in sleeping, accompanied by on-going fatigue. Significant fatigue the day after a workout. Chest pains (immediately consult a doctor).

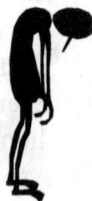

Excessive exercise can be dangerous to certain types of people such as tense, impatient, anger-oriented people; and especially those who are a strongly Type A personality.

Exercise may aggravate their tension, rather than relax them, as it does most people. As in all other aspects of health, moderation is the important key.

Recreational sports, while valuable for recreational purposes and for some degree of fitness, are not as valuable as a designed exercise program which includes a continuous, rhythmic, controlled overload and range of movement. Most competition sports are an invitation to over-exertion, and do not have the continuous rhythmic movements necessary for optimal conditioning. The ideal method of participating in highly competitive sports is to train for them, using a designed exercise program which prepares the participants for the maximum exertion anticipated in the sport. Participation in sports is an excellent motivator for following an exercise program.

An exercise program should always begin with a 2 to 10 minute warm-up such as gentle calisthenics, jogging in place, etc. Then do some stretching movements, but **do not attempt to stretch <u>cold</u> muscles, ligaments, and tendons**. Warm up before stretching. **Do not bounce your stretches**, and increase your stretches gradually. Many people find themselves surprised at how rapidly stretching progresses in just a few days.

It is possible to maintain a high level of fitness, vigor and vitality as we age, even into our seventies and eighties, and well beyond. The keys are to recognize the fact that we will slow down some, and that we are somewhat more prone to muscle, tendon, joint, and bone injuries as time goes on. The benefits of exercise have been shown to occur at all ages however, and the very act of exercise greatly reduces the chance of bone injury by stimulating bone formation to keep the bones strong. So we merely need to make a few changes in our exercise program as we age.

We can avoid injuries better as we age by emphasizing less violent, more rhythmic movements - especially in our sports. The benefits of appropriate exercise at any age far outweigh the risk of injury.

The greatest "youth pill" discovered so far, is strenuous exercise. Vigorous, strenuous, enthusiastic exercise. And it really appears to work as a youth pill. When a guy meets a girl - especially when an older guy meets a younger girl that he likes a lot, what's the first thing that he does? He starts running, he does push-ups, and so on. And what does a girl do? Of course, the first thing that she does is to watch what she eats a little more carefully (or a lot more carefully). But she will also do her leg lifts, her sit-ups, her lady push-ups, her aerobics, and perhaps her running, with greater diligence.

They do these exercises - and others - because they really do promote attractiveness and feelings of youthfulness. The stimulation caused by strenuous exercise generates such great circulation of the blood, that every part of the body is flushed clean and clear, and then receives a flood of fresh nutrients and oxygen.

Along with nutrients and oxygen though, come several life and youth-giving chemicals that stimulate new life, vigor, strength, sexuality, and positive thinking. Positive thinking is a proven benefit of certain specific chemicals - especially endorphins (a naturally produced opiate) produced by the brain, as a direct result of exercising.

Exercise programs are a planned method of creating activity in each and every part of the body, thus assuring that every area of the body receives the circulation needed to flush itself out, and to deliver the nutrients, oxygen, and chemicals that bring health, youthfulness, and attractiveness.

Just the desire to remain healthy enough to stay out of hospitals and be fully active and able to do all of the things that you like to do is enough motivation to work out regularly.

The social benefits of being very youthful and attractive from working out regularly, although secondary in importance, are also pleasurable and rewarding.

Everyone can, and must, exercise. The very young must work out to develop their abilities, and keep their health and youthfulness (many of us have seen how fast it can fade), and to form good exercise habits early. Older men and women must work out to maintain or regain a healthy, youthful, and attractive condition.

The proof of the benefits of working out for older people who have never worked out is shown most dramatically in the story that came from the research center of a major California university some years ago. The researchers started, as an experiment, with a woman approaching her 90's, who had never been involved in exercise, and who was so bent over and stiff that she could barely shuffle across the street. After just two years of working with her, she was standing upright, and was not only competing in the Senior Olympics, but she actually won the 1500 meter run two years in a row!

Cardiologists concluded some time ago that after a heart attack, even a very severe one, the patient will ideally be put on an exercise program that should develop into strenuous exercise and running.

The fact is that modern research has shown clearly that one of the biggest causes of "aging", and the "illnesses" of "old age" are to a great degree a direct result of people becoming less and less active as their lives progress. We know that there is actually no illness, and no deterioration of any kind in man that is just a result of the passage of time. Deterioration as a result of inactivity occurs at every age, but happens faster after we are fully grown and mature if people become less and less active.

The truth about exercise is that we need more and more exercise as our lives progress, not less and less, as some of us were brought up to believe. The life forces, which we inherited, grow, develop, and mature, keep us healthy, attractive, and youthful only until we are grown, developed, and matured. Then we must take over the maintenance and development of our own health, youthfulness, and attractiveness.

The bottom line is: Use It Or Lose It; and this applies to all of our faculties: physical, mental, and emotional.

Face Exercises

A West Coast woman, considering massive plastic surgery at the age of 46, was introduced by a research foundation to the possible benefits of improved health and beauty, through improved self care. She embarked on a campaign of facial and body exercise, improved nutrition, and self-massage of the face.

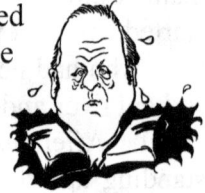

While using these self-improvement methods, her attitude toward herself changed dramatically.

As a direct result of her efforts, she had only very minor plastic surgery. When an old classmate and she had a picture taken together, they both commented that, instead of looking 5 years older than her age, she now looked 10 years younger than her classmate. It has often been said that beauty is 20% nature, and 80% self-care.

Only in recent years has it been commonly recognized that the shape of the face, the fullness of the features, and the attractiveness of the facial expressions are dependent on the condition of the facial muscles. When the facial muscles, through lack of use, become smaller the cheeks and the eyes appear sunken, and the skin, no longer filled out by full facial muscles, sags and wrinkles. Obviously, this gives the appearance of advanced aging.

These problems can be alleviated by regular exercise of all of the facial muscles, by proper nutrition - especially vitamins C and D, and by feeding and protecting the skin from the weather with skin lotions.

If performed regularly, The Face Exercises can help to keep the face looking full, well-formed, full of personality, more wrinkle-free, and highly attractive.
1) Make funny faces of all kinds, for about 1 1/2 minutes, bringing the neck muscles into play.
2) Fill both cheeks with air, then force all of the air back and forth from one cheek to the
     other, for about one minute.
3) Wet the lips, and rub them one against the other as though applying lipstick. Do this for about 1/2 minute. This will help keep the lips full, and avoid the aged look of too-thin lips.
4) Yoga gives us the "Lion" face exercise: Open the eyes wide, stick the tongue out as far as possible, and lean the head forward slightly. Hold for about 20 seconds. Do this exercise 3 times.

The Face Exercises can eliminate some bagging under the eyes, wrinkled and sagging skin, and bring circulation to the entire face. As with other parts of the body, atrophy is the face's worst enemy. The Face Exercise stimulates and revitalizes the "frozen" areas of the face.

Eye Exercises

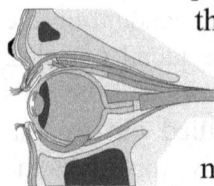

Some vision problems are simply the result of weakness of the eye muscles, arising from an insufficient range of visual activity. Our daily habits sometimes cause us to use our eyes only in certain ways, and often these ways do not utilize the entire range of our visual potential. The unused ranges of our visual field then atrophy, causing degeneration of those areas of focus. So, in order to maintain or regain the strength and ability to see well now and in the future, we must care for our eyes just as we must feed our stomachs and breathe.

These Eye Exercises will stimulate and energize all of the muscles which move the eyes so that healthy, comfortable eyes are maintained or regained. Naturally, healthy and stimulated eyes will be more attractive eyes.

The Eye Exercises may be performed sitting, standing, or lying down.

1) Holding the head perfectly still, look up as high as possible without raising the eyebrows; and hold it for 5 seconds; then look left 5 seconds; then down 5 seconds; then right 5 seconds. Do this twice.

2) Rotate the eyes: Look up; left; down; right; then up again. Do this 3 times. Pause a moment; then reverse the direction: Look up; right; down; left; then up again. Do this 3 times.

3) To exercise the muscles which focus the eyes: Go to a window: look into the distance as far as you can see; then gradually look closer and closer until you are looking at the tip of your nose; then gradually look away until you are again looking at your distant starting point. Do this 10 times.

These exercises, done daily, may help to resolve some eye problems, and can help to keep your eyes in good health.

Meditation

The simpler the meditation is, the more beneficial it will be. It is primarily a time for self-contact, self-realization, and a conscious alignment of personal priorities. The fact that everything follows the mind is the basis for the statement that, "If one sets one's mind, most things are possible".

If one continues to meditate, the objectives of the meditation must be realized. It cannot be otherwise. Decide, before meditating, on some TOPICS on which you wish to meditate. They can be anything in your life, but must focus on you.

Meditation Suggestions

The Meditation is best done at the same time every day. Get into any comfortable position, in a quiet place. Try to keep the mind on the inner feelings of self, and on the TOPICS of the MEDITATION. Try not to let the mind wander in a disorganized manner.

1) Establish contact with your inner being; the body; the mind; then the emotions. Listen to yourself, and get to know yourself better.

2) Consider the TOPICS you selected: TOPIC 1; then Topic 2; then Topic 3; then Topic 4, etc.

The meditation can last for 3 minutes, or for hours; but you might want to keep it to about 5 to15 minutes. Before you start, set a time limit to meditate.

Everyone should consult their doctor before following any exercise program.

Carl Bourhenne's Personal Workout

I began developing my workout in 1955, and have been studying and improving it every year.

My workout has been carefully designed to work every part of the body from the top of the head to the tips of the toes.

Every body part that is not exercised regularly will deteriorate over time and will cease to function normally.

The old adage, "Use it or lose it" is true for each and every part of the body. Another way to say it is, "Move it or lose it" and if we don't, it will gradually fade away.

Exercises for my workout are from such sources as the Canadian Mounted Police workout, Yoga, T'ai Ch'i Chuan, and Arnold Schwarzenegger's workout.

I have studied the significant exercise programs in various countries over these years, and continue to watch new trends as they develop. I have tested and modified it over the years, along with newer concepts from reliable sources, public and private.

This Work-out can be your ideal, efficient, lifetime exercise program. It consists of the movements and activities of stretching, weight training, running and aerobic activity, which our bodies, minds, and emotions need in order to:

1) Exercise every muscle in the body.
2) Provide circulatory and cardio-vascular conditioning.
3) Develop balance and coordination.

For details of how to perform these routines I recommend,

Carl Bourhenne's Workout Video.

Note that all reliable sources strongly recommend weight lifting as par t of any exercise program, since it is absolutely necessary to put pressure on the bones for them to \stay strong.

The reason I have two workout sections is that we must not work the same muscles hard two days in a row, as they need time to rebuild between workouts, except for the abdominal muscles and the calf muscles which are slightly different in makeup.

"I follow this workout religiously, and I have done so for the last 63 years. At the age of 82, I am very, very pleased that I actually have."

I have no health problems, I take no medications, I am sexually active most days, and my blood pressure, cholesterol and sugar are normal.

I want very much to be able to say the same thing when I am 110 years old and over.

<u>Every movement or one like it that you leave out will result in one or more of your body parts steadily deteriorating for the rest of your life.</u>

<u>And yes, it's a lot to do, but the results are AMAZING for your health, and your long life.</u>

Carl Bourhenne's Personal Workout

WARM-UPS
WARM-UP <u>MONDAY</u> Thru <u>SATURDAY</u>

KNEE LIFTS (20 ea leg twice), RUN OR STATIONARY BIKE (At least 15 minutes) W/FINGER CURLS (100) KNEE LIFTS (20 ea. leg twice).

SHOULDER ROTATIONS (5 each side 2x),

FACE EXERCISES: Lion (20); Cheeks: Side-to-side (20); Cheeks: Up-and-down: (20); Lips (30)
EYE EXERCISES: Side-to-side (5); up-and-down (5), Rotate (5) Eyes Focus Far/Near,

NECK: Forward-back (10), Side-to side (5), Rotate (5 each direction)
WAIST: Lean way forward (10), Lean way backward (10), Rotate at waist (5 each direction)
HEAD & SHOULDER TWIST (10 each way)

CALF LIFTS (15)
BUTTOCK LIFTS (10 each leg); GLUTE SQUEEZES (10 slow, 10 fast, 10 slow)
PROSTATE EXERCISES (Kegel), (10 fast, 10 slow, 10 fast), Light Massage
KNEE BENDS (20); STANDING LEG STRETCHES (10 each leg)

SIT-UPS (15); LEG-UPS (5); SCISSORS (10); DONKEY KICKS (10); BUTTOCK LIFTS (10); PUSH-UPS (5); BUTTOCK UP-DRIVES (10), SITTING LEG STRETCHES

BALANCE MOVEMENT (20 count each leg)

WED & SAT: TOE CURLS (100 each foot); MEDITATION (5-15 Min)

LIFTING WEIGHTS

MONDAY and THURSDAY (Chest & Back)

BENCH PRESS: Barbell (8-12) FLAT; Dumbbells (8-12) FLAT; Dumbbells (8-12) INCLINE; Dumbbells (8-12 DECLINE)

BUTTERFLIES: INCLINE (8-12); DECLINE (8-12); FLAT (8-12)

LAT PULL-DOWNS (8-12)

ONE-ARM UP-ROWS (8-12; SEATED ROWS (8-12); T-BAR UP-ROWS (8-12)

TOE CURLS (100 each foot); MEDITATION (5-15 Min)

TUESDAY and FRIDAY (Shoulders, Arms, and Legs)

LATERAL RAISES: Front (8-12)
SHOULDER SHRUGS: (8-12)
CALVES (15)

BENCH: BUTTOCK CURLS (8-12); LEG CURLS (8-12); LEG EXTENSIONS (8-12)

SQUATS (8-12)

WRIST CURLS (8-12)
TRICEPS: Reverse Curls (8-12) Triceps bar (8-12); Reverse Push-ups (10)
BICEPS: REVERSE CURLS (8-12); Dumbbells (8-12); Barbell (8-12)
TOE CURLS (100 each foot); MEDITATION: (5-15 Min)

Carl Bourhenne, MA
Gerontologist

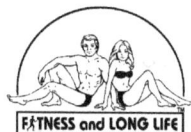

How To Live
The Longest Life Possible

Weight Management

Permanent Weight Control

Permanent weight control can only be accomplished by **permanent lifestyle changes**. That is why **DIETS DON'T WORK**. If the things that you are doing to lose weight are not permanent lifestyle changes the results are not likely to be permanent, either.

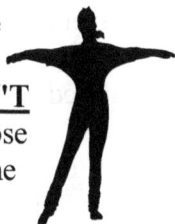

As many of us who have tried several types of diets for weight loss have found out, but perhaps not realized that,

DIETS DO NOT WORK!

The ONLY thing that works is,

PERMANENT LIFESTYLE CHANGES.

To those who have never really thought about it, this will come as a startling statement that may be a little hard to accept, but if you are overweight you are living proof that diets do not work, because you have probably used several of them yourself. **People in the United States alone spent $33 billion on diets in 1996, and 95% of them failed.** The other 5% must have made permanent lifestyle changes, or they also would have regained the weight.

Jean Mayer, the renowned nutritionist, refers to these up and down weight loss methods as the "rhythm method of girth control". The fact is that a temporary diet is not a lasting solution to an overweight condition. An overweight condition is the result of a combination of factors including, but perhaps not limited to heredity, and psychological, sociological, and biological conditions. These conditions may include such factors as metabolism, hypo-activity (insufficient exercise), escapism, frustration, insecurity, and others.

The long term solution to weight management is a permanent behavior modification program that includes addressing the reasons and the occasions of eating more than is required for the maintenance of one's desirable weight.

Few of us have inherited the genetic predisposition to meet the ideals portrayed in TV commercials and billboard advertisements. It is important that we accept the body style which we inherited, and appreciate ourselves for who and what we are. Nevertheless, we all do have some control over how we look as regards our weight. There are two main reasons for controlling our weight. We all want to have a pleasing appearance, and to be healthy.

While contemporary society may be overly infatuated with a slender appearance, overweight is nevertheless associated with several major diseases and causes of death, such as the following. <u>Hypertension</u> (high blood pressure): It is known to be a significant cause of stroke, heart disease, and kidney disease. <u>Heart Disease</u>:

Overweight is responsible for one-fourth of deaths from heart disease in the United States, especially for people who are 30% or more overweight. <u>Diabetes</u>: Overweight contributes significantly to the development of diabetes, which may lead to heart attack, stroke, blindness, and atherosclerosis. <u>Cancer</u>: Some research shows that women who are overweight have a higher incidence of cancers of the uterus, breast, gall bladder, and pancreas; and if overweight since adolescence, incidences of endometrial (uterine lining) cancer is 75% greater.

Problems associated with overweight are many because most every facet of life is affected. Disadvantages are felt in one's self-esteem, emotional, social, as well as one's vocational life.

Some Major Considerations In Weight Management Are:

Speed of eating: When we eat rapidly our appetite regulating mechanism does not have time to signal satiety. Indeed, when so abused, this mechanism may switch off, in time.

Heavy eating late in the day: In most people, this can be a major factor in weight gain. <u>Eat Late, Gain Weight!</u>

Junk food habits: High calorie, low nutrient foods are habituating, and more is required to satisfy hunger.

The first step in a good weight control program is to develop a Behavior Modification program to make permanent changes in eating and drinking habits. The starting move is to observe when, what, where, with whom, why (if possible), and how we eat. Make notes for a week on each of these issues. At the end of the week, look at your notes and draw some conclusions that can help you to make some decisions for changing your eating, exercise, and social habits. It could be helpful to get some professional help.

While eating less calories than we burn up is one perspective on weight control, the flip side is burning up more calories than we eat by increasing our activity level. The best way to do this is to increase our level of daily exercise.

Some considerations in developing an exercise program are:

In order to lose weight you <u>must</u> exercise. The reason is that the body will first give up weight in water, then in perceived unused muscle. If you use your muscles each day <u>then</u> the body will give up fat.

The <u>type of exercise</u> you select should be one you enjoy, and that fits into your lifestyle. Exercising at <u>the same time every day</u> creates a routine which becomes a regular part of your schedule, making the exercise somewhat easier to get into.

The <u>type of exercise</u> is less important than consistency and frequency. <u>Aerobic exercises,</u> that is continuous, rhythmic exercise lasting thirty minutes or longer, are the most beneficial. Walking, swimming, jogging, bicycling, and rowing are among the best.

<u>Avoid shots, pills, miracle diets, and other super-quick weight loss fads.</u>

Always consult your doctor before beginning any new strenuous programs.

The most valuable guidelines for successful weight control include these:

1. The menu for your weight loss program must be identical to the menu that you will use after you reach your desirable weight. The only differences for weight loss

are increase in exercise combined with a reduction in the amount of higher calorie types of foods. Do not eliminate any foods from your menu during weight loss.

2. Eat a good breakfast, including a complete protein.
3. Do not skip meals, and eat them at about the same time every day.
4. Eat moderate portions, and never take seconds.
5. Eat larger portions of vegetables, and smaller portions of high calorie foods.
6. Snacks (2 or 3) at regular intervals between meals are O.K., but they must be nutritious items such as fruits, vegetables, or dry cereals.
7. Chew your food well, and eat slowly. You will feel more satisfied without getting overly full. **Never fill your stomach.**
8. Have specific places at home, work, and school where you do nothing but eat. Do not eat while doing something else, such as watching TV. Break associations between
   eating and doing other things, especially recreating.
9. Never eat because of depression, loneliness, anxiety, or for escape. Turn to non food or drink activities such as social relationships, sports or games, creative activity, work, academic activity, or some other non food or drink activity which you enjoy.
10. Keep clearly in mind the way you want to look and feel.

To attain and maintain your desirable weight then, first decide exactly what your desirable weight is, and then **plan your permanent lifetime weight control program**. Get some help if needed, and follow your plan enthusiastically, passionately and consistently.

Remember, after you reach your desirable weight, <u>the only difference between the losing phase and the maintaining phase should be a slight increase in the amount of each type of food that you eat, with no change</u>

in the types of food eaten. Your body needs the same kinds of nutrition in both phases, just less calories and perhaps more exercise. Eat some of everything that you want to include in your permanent menu, both for weight loss and, as importantly, to form new eating and drinking habits. Practicing the permanent eating and drinking habits while losing weight is the key to making the weight loss permanent. The main reason that "diets" don't work is because they don't let you practice and form your new eating and drinking habits.

The No Stress Diet

The following "diet" offers insight into some common sub-conscious notions about eating and dieting.

Breakfast
- 1/2 Grapefruit
- 1 Slice Whole Wheat Toast
- 8 oz. Skim Milk

Lunch
- 4 OZ. Lean Broiled Chicken Breast
- 1 Cup Steamed Zucchini
- 1 Oreo Cookie
- Herb Tea

Mid-Afternoon Snack
- Rest of the Package of Oreos
- 1 Quart Rocky Road Ice Cream
- 1 Jar Hot Fudge

Dinner
- 2 Loaves Garlic Bread
- Large Pepperoni and Mushroom Pizza
- Large Pitcher of Beer
- 3 Milky Way Candy Bars
- Entire Frozen Cheesecake - Eaten directly from the freezer

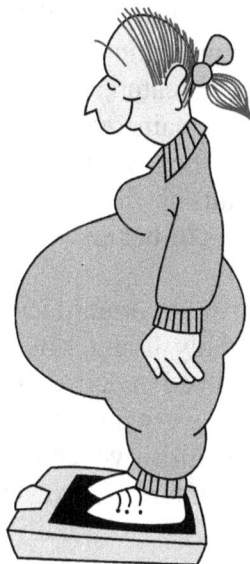

Diet Tips

1. If no one sees you eat it, it has no calories. If you drink a diet soda with a candy bar, they cancel each other out.
2. When eating with someone else, calories don't count if you both eat the same amount.
3. Foods used for medicinal purposes NEVER count; such as, Hot Chocolate, Brandy, Toast, and Cheesecake.
4. If you fatten up everyone else around you, then you look thinner.
5. Movie related foods don't count because they are simply part of the entire entertainment experience and not a part of one's personal fuel; such as Milk Duds, Popcorn and Butter, and Junior Mints.
6. Whatever your favorite food is, it's a **Negative Food** (chewing it burns up more calories than it contains).

** Take this "diet" with a LARGE grain of salt.

We have all seen how overweight people tend to look 10 to 20 years older than they are. And we have also seen people lose weight, and appear ten years younger. Excess weight not only makes people look older, but it can cause bagging under the eyes, wrinkled and sagging skin, and other unhealthy and unattractive features. These features become more and more permanent the longer we remain overweight. Also, fat people may die younger than they would if they were to stay in a slim condition, as a result of the extreme physical and sometimes emotional stress of being overweight.

An important factor in weight control is a high motivation in daily living. Being excited about the things that we are involved in daily, and being excited about the people we deal with every day can cause us to keep ourselves in the healthy and attractive condition necessary to coordinate with our own interests. Anyone who is less than excited about what they do in their daily life, or with whom they associate might make whatever changes are needed to allow them to begin doing something they enjoy doing for a living, for recreation, and for a social life. There are never any valid reasons for not pursuing the life that we want. There are no barriers that large, or hurdles that high. And anyone who is having difficulty coming up with the ideas to do this should speak with a friend, or a counselor. This is your real life. It is not a dress rehearsal. If the way that you are living your life isn't exciting, interesting, and fun, you might have difficulty changing your weight. The change is in your hands only.

Exercise by itself is not a long term method of weight control or weight loss. Moderate exercise when combined with eating control causes faster weight loss, but exercising too strenuously while dieting can be dangerous.

The only cause of weight loss is burning up more calories than we take in, pure and simple. Ever notice the overweight pro football player? Do you know how murderously strenuous their daily exercise routine is? Some of them are overweight. **Those who are overweight are simply eating more than they burn up.**

Depending on frame, level of activity, and age (we burn up less calories as we grow older). The "average" man requires about 20 calories per day for each pound of body weight; and the "average" woman requires about 17 calories per day for each pound of body weight. The difference between the heaviest and the lightest frame are negligible, when considered with other off-setting personal factors.

A woman who weighs 100 lb. requires about 1700 calories per day to maintain her weight: (100 x 17 = 1700 calories).

Recent research shows that life expectancy can be dramatically improved by reducing that number.

A man who weighs 170 lb. requires about 3400 calories per day to maintain his body weight: (170 x 20 = 3400).

Recent research shows that life expectancy can be dramatically improved by reducing that number.

Of course, the actual exact number of calories that you require must be determined by you, by trial and by observing the results. This is, however, an ideal starting number, and we're sure you'll like the results.

Perhaps the one factor that determines our weight more than any other, is **when we eat**. What we eat early in the day our faster metabolism tends to burn up, and then we begin burning up fat. What we eat later in the day we tend to store as fat; especially if we go to sleep without having burned it all up.

So, the first thing that must be done to set up a weight maintenance program, or a weight loss program is to determine the number of calories you burn up each day:

Women multiply your ideal body weight by 17.

Men multiply your ideal body weight by 20.

If you are already at your ideal weight, then this is the approximate number of calories you need to eat each day. Remember, though, this will probably not be exact for you, and you'll have to adjust this number as you watch the results over a few month's time.

Never eat until your stomach is completely full. The entire system becomes congested and clogged, putting stress on the system, and causing damage to the body. Eat slowly enough to foresee the point of satisfaction, and thus avoid over-eating. Remember, the stomach continues to fill up for some time after we stop eating, because the system must continue to add digestive juices to process the food just eaten. So we must leave a little room in our stomachs for the addition of these digestive juices. If we pack the food into our stomach too much, the digestive juices cannot penetrate into the food at a normal rate, and we are left with both a digesting, and a comfort problem.

You can see from your figures that you can realistically expect to lose about 1½ to 2 pounds per week. Remember, if you start out knowing that you are actually only losing about 1½ to 2 pounds per week of fat, you shouldn't become discouraged after that first week or two of losing 5 to 8 pounds per week of water. If you are exercising, you will be adding muscle, which weighs about twice as much as fat, so allow for that exchange when you weigh yourself. **Don't weigh yourself more than twice per week.**

To figure out how long it will take you to reach your ideal weight, then, determine how many pounds you must lose, subtract 5 to 10 (for the initial quick water weight loss), then multiply by 3 (about a third of a pound per day). This will tell you about haw many days it will take you to be your ideal weight. For example: If you want to weigh 120 lb., but you weigh 140, then you want to lose 20 lb.

20 minus 5 = 15 lb., so multiply that by 3 (3 x 15 = 45), and you can see that you should allow yourself about 45 days to lose the 20 lb. of excess weight that you carry.

Now, look at your calendar and mark the day you will be at your ideal weight. It is important to remember, if you do have excess fat on your body, that you didn't accumulate it in a week and you won't lose it in a week, either.

<u>For every 3500 calories that you eat in excess of your need, you gain one pound. And you must burn up 3500 calories more than you eat, to lose one pound.</u>

Everyone who starts a weight loss program immediately loses five to eight pounds, usually in the first one to three days. Obviously, this cannot possibly be all fat, since you would have to burn up 17,500 calories to lose 5 lb. (3500 x 5 = 17,500). If you normally burn 2,000 calories per day, and your weight loss program is 1,200 calories, you will be reducing by 2,400 calories in three days - less than 1 pound. Even if you fasted for five days, you'd burn up 4,000 calories; not even near the 17,500 needed to burn up 5 pounds.

So as you've probably already figured out, the largest part of your first three to five days of weight loss is water. Don't be discouraged when your loss of pounds slows down dramatically after the first three to five days.

Begin now to look at yourself, and to think of yourself as being your ideal weight, and it can soon be true. By the way, along with good motivation you should try to arrange freedom from major frustrations. Major frustrations are those which arise from neglecting to pursue the things in life that are really important to you; such as a particular kind of work; a certain kind of lifestyle; certain social activities; or a port or hobby that you have always wanted to participate in; etc. So in order to be slim, you may have to change jobs, start your own business, change your domestic situation, take some lessons or classes to facilitate the changes; or simply adopt new attitudes toward your present situations.

Gaining Weight

There are some important factors to consider when gaining weight. Three of the factors are involved in an underweight condition: heredity, eating habits, and exercise habits. Some often controllable habits which contribute to underweight include undereating, nervous tension, lack of muscle developing exercise, nervous tension, and hyperactivity. Gaining weight must involve planned, consistent program, which deals with the observance of new habits.

The successful weight gain program will include increased calorie intake (mostly carbohydrates), moderate exercise, and stress control.

It is important to note that high protein and high fat diets can be dangerous. Also, while muscle can be added to specific body areas by exercising those muscles, it is not possible to add fat to designated areas.

To gain weight, maintain top nutritional standards, and do not smoke or drink coffee with caffeine. In addition, eat all of the whole grain products, fruits, baked potatoes, honey, and nuts that you wish.

Strenuous exercise can help, if you feed yourself accordingly.

Carl Bourhenne, MA
Gerontologist

FITNESS and LONG LIFE

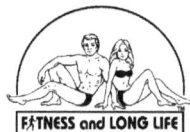

How To Live
The Longest Life Possible

Nutrition

I will begin this section with a summary of **some of the most important nutritional guidelines:**

1. Make your food primarily vegetables and fruits so that you eat a primarily plant-based diet.
2. For protein, eat mostly fish, chicken, and other low fat sources. Avoid eating too much protein, as research shows that **excess protein causes rapid aging**.
3. Eat a wide variety of vegetables. There are seven colors of vegetables, and each contains its own nutrients and phytonutrients.
4. **Remember well that no vitamin pills contain the phytonutrients critically necessary for your health that are contained only in vegetables and fruits**.
5. Carbohydrates can comprise 60% of our calories: 40% from vegetables, grains, breads, and legumes; and 20% from fruit.

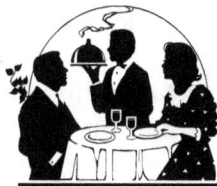

6. **Fat should comprise 25% <u>or less</u> of the daily calorie intake**. Saturated fats should be half as much as mono-unsaturated and poly-unsaturated fats combined. Prefer Poly-unsaturated fats.

7. Eat no more than 65 grams of protein per day (should be no more than 10% to 15% of the total calories.) **Excess protein causes rapid aging**.

8. Cholesterol intake must be less than 300 Mg. per day. One egg yolk contains 250 Mg.

9. Eat sufficient Fiber, but not to excess since **excess fiber flushes needed nutrients**.

10. **Avoid refined sugars**, which promote free radicals and cause other health problems, and have no nutritional value.

11. Watch out for sodium by reading labels, and hold salt usage to 1 teaspoon per day. Natural foods have adequate salt. **Adding salt to food is not necessary**.

12. Avoid nitrites, and any meats that are charcoaled or burnt, and do not cook meats, especially pork, at 300ø or more. **All of these create nitrosomines which are powerful carcinogens (cancer-causing agents)**. Do not eat grains or nuts with mold, which generate aflatoxins, also the most powerful carcinogens.

13. Drink about **8 glasses of quality water per day**.

14. Try to **breathe deeply** and regularly throughout the day.

15. **Get a little sunlight**, but use the recommended type of **sunscreen**, not just PABA (See, LIGHT).

16. **Do not eat raw eggs**, or products containing raw eggs. **Raw eggs may have salmonella**.

Nutrition Basics

There is, perhaps, more misinformation regarding nutrition and its effects on our health and long life, than on any other aspect of health and long life. In addition, the reliable information on

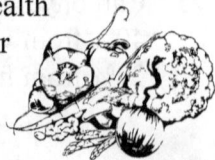

70

nutrition may be the most confusing of any other aspect of health and long life. The reason for this confusion could well reside in the fact that nutrition itself is a very complex body of knowledge. **We need 50 nutrients** for health, and to continue our life processes. These 50 nutrients each contributes in its own way; and in addition, they interact with one another in various ways. By thinking of these nutrients in groups, we can more easily get a grasp of how they help keep us healthy and alive.

The 50 nutrients can be thought of as 6 easy to remember groups:

Proteins, Carbohydrates, Fats, Vitamins, Minerals, Water & Air

If we list the amino acids (the building blocks of Proteins), the Carbohydrates, the types of Fats, the Vitamins, the Minerals, and Water & Air, we arrive at about 50 Essential Nutrients.

It is even simpler, though, to think of these needed nutrients in terms of their sources - mainly our food. The factor which makes this approach very easy to understand is the fact that our foods, with all of the 50 nutrients, can be divided into **only four food groups** which contain all of the nutrients we need for a healthy Long Life, youthful and attractive.

We are all quite familiar with these foods, and know them as **The Four Food Groups:**
1. **The Meat Group** (all animal foods, including fish and poultry and their eggs; peas, dried beans and other legumes; and nuts.)
2. **Milk And Milk Products**
3. **Fruits And Vegetables**

4. **Breads And Cereals** (Including spaghetti, noodles, macaroni, rice, and the like.)

We need all of the 50 nutrients in these four food groups to be healthy, and to live as long a life as we can, youthful and attractive. These nutrients provide materials for the manufacture of bones, skin, hair, muscles, hormones, and enzymes; as well as providing fuel for all body processes.

The result of too little nutrition, or too much nutrition are surpassed by the results of too much non-nutritive food.

Some foods contain all four of the food groups, such as pizza; and some belong to none of the food groups, and serve only as condiments or calorie additives (sugar, condiments, spreads, dressings, etc.).

Coloring, Preservatives, Additives, Flavorings
These all call for special comment. First of all, how do we know what of these, if any, are in the foods we purchase?

Since 1973, enacted laws require that any food which has been *enriched* or *fortified*, or that makes any nutritional claim, must be labeled with seven types of nutritional information. (*Enrichment* refers to the process where specific nutrients - niacin, thiamin, riboflavin, and iron - lost in processing are restored to the equivalent levels in the natural product; and *fortification* refers to the addition of one or more nutrients not originally present in that food.)
The seven types of nutritional information required on these food labels are:

Serving size, servings per container, calories per serving, protein, carbohydrates, fat, and the percentage of RDA (Recommended Dietary Allowances) for the essential nutrients: protein, vitamins A, D, niacin thiamin, riboflavin, calcium, and iron.

72

An "*" next to the vitamin or mineral indicates that the food contains less than 2% of the U.S. **RDA**. The **RDA's** are reviewed for revision every five years, and are the estimated best quantities for persons with the highest physiological requirement; so eating the **RDA** level assures anyone of meeting all of their nutritional needs.

While it is true that foods would be much more expensive to the consumer without preservatives (there would be enormous amounts of spoilage); and while some preservatives prevent some food-borne potentially fatal diseases, like salmonella and botulism; it is, nevertheless important to look at additives and preservatives over-all.

Some are actually nutrients (some synthetic) which enhance or replace certain vitamins or minerals.

Preservatives, *antioxidants*, and *bleaches* delay, or even prevent spoilage. Additives such as *stabilizers*, *thickeners*, and *emulsifiers* improve consistency, texture, and uniformity. Sourness and tartness are controlled by *acidulants*, and *sequestrants* keep foods from appearing cloudy. *Humectants* preserve moisture in foods, while *firming agents* prevent softening of fruits and vegetables, and *flavoring agents* are used.

Studies from both independent and government sources show that **some additives are not safe.** Regardless of the debated effects of the above additives and preservatives, two other kinds demand special attention: nitrite curing agents, and chemical coloring.

For example, **nitrites, which are used to control food color (especially in meats) are known to convert to the powerful cancer-causing agents nitrosomines when cooked over 300°, or while in the human body.**

Also, one of the most used food coloring agents - **Red Dye II** - has been found to be carcinogenic (cancer-causing) in laboratory animals. Alarmingly, since expiration of the proof-of-safety requirement in 1962, the FDA has not required completion of the necessary safety studies. This fact is especially disturbing because most food colorings are coal-tar colors, which have been implicated in many serious diseases including cancer. Equally alarming is the fact that the scientists who test food additives are paid by the food industry itself; so, obviously we must wonder what protection the consumer will realize from these studies.

Nutritional information of special importance to many comes from the subject of malnutrition. It is highly significant that malnutrition means "bad nutrition", which includes both under-nutrition and over-nutrition. "Over-nutrition" causes such diseases as heart disease, cancer, and diabetes in those pre-disposed to it. About 10% of the U.S. population suffer the many diseases caused by malnourishment because of too little food. Another 10% - the upper income group - are also malnourished because of poor food choice, especially of too much high calorie fatty foods, sweets, and salt. This over-nutrition leads to heart disease; cancer of the colon, breast, and prostate gland; and gallstones.

A popular myth in our society is that we must consume large amounts of protein. Many of the foods we eat contain protein, so we do not need to pay special attention to protein intake in order to assure adequate amounts in our diet. Quite the contrary.

Recent research shows that too much protein intake causes rapid aging and diabetes. It is important to note that one of the popular fad diets for weight loss is especially dangerous. Potassium deficiencies caused by low-carbohydrate diets can result in heart irregularity, which can be fatal.

The 6 Types Of Nutrients

Proteins, Carbohydrates, Fats, Vitamins, Minerals, Water & Air

1) Proteins: The 23 Amino Acids are the Building Blocks of the body, and are what proteins are made of. Amino Acids are chemicals composed of carbon, hydrogen, oxygen, nitrogen, and sulfur; arranged in various ways. The **RDA** is 65 grams of Protein per day. Since the average American consumes 106 grams per day, they take in far more than is needed. The excess is either converted to glucose and burned as energy, or converted to glycogen, then stored as fat. This proves to be an expensive source of energy, and too much protein tends to elevate urea levels in the blood.

Protein of plant origin (vegetables and grains) is almost always incomplete protein; but plant proteins can be combined with one another, or with animal proteins to form complete protein. **Some such combinations are:** Cereal with milk; macaroni with cheese; rice with beans; beans with corn tortillas.

Protein is necessary for the construction of muscles, hair, teeth, nails, bones, nerve cells, hemoglobin and enzymes. Proteins are what RNA and DNA are made of (DNA is the substance which constitutes our genes, and RNA is the transcription of DNA for the repair and reproduction of our body parts and functions.

Severe protein deficiency causes "kwashiorkor" - a condition which affects children, primarily. The result can be slow growth, bloated stomachs, severe mental retardation, apathy, and pigment changes, causing a slightly purplish appearance. In the young or the mature adult, even small deficiencies of protein for a time can result in irritability, reduced antibody production, and fatigue. The effects are reduced ability to fight disease and heal wounds. If the deficiency continues, anemia and liver disorders may result.

Proteins are the highly important "building blocks" of the cells. They are the materials that the cell is actually made of. Just as a brick house is made of bricks, a cell is made of proteins. However, the body accepts only "complete proteins". **Complete proteins are proteins that are made up of certain parts, called "<u>amino acids</u>". So, the body will only build cells from complete proteins, made up of the following amino acids: <u>Tryptophane</u>, <u>Threonine</u>, <u>Phenylalanine</u>, <u>Lysine</u>, <u>Valine</u>, <u>Isoleucine</u>, <u>Methionine</u>, and <u>Leucine</u>.**

Moreover, **these 8 <u>Essential</u> Amino Acids** must be in a certain relation to each other. For each 1 part of tryptophane, there must also be: 2 parts threonine; 2 parts phenylalanine, 3 parts each of lysine, valine, isoleucine, and methionine; and 3.4 parts leucine.

There are other amino acids which the body requires, bringing the total to 23; but it can manufacture all of the others from these 8, which it cannot manufacture.

Now, unless you are a micro-biologist, you are wondering how in the world you are going to know how to provide your body with these needs. **It's really quite simple: Just eat the foods that contain these "complete proteins", daily. These foods are, in order of their value: Eggs, Milk, Fish, Meat, Poultry, Cheese, Most seeds, nuts, grains, vegetables, and legumes.**

The National Research Council recommends a daily intake of 0.42 grams of protein for each pound of body weight. So, if you divide your weight by 2, you will have the approximate number of grams of protein you need each day. All excess protein is either burned up as energy, or stored as fat. 1 gram of protein provides about 4 calories. Since every 3,500 excess calories you consume adds 1 pound of fat to your body, every 875 grams of protein you take in but don't burn up adds 1 pound of fat to the body.

So, it is vital for a healthy Long Life, youthful and attractive, to get sufficient "complete protein" to sustain cell life and cell reproduction. It is also important not to consume excess calories, since excess fat on the body inhibits healthy cell life.

2) Carbohydrates: There are 3 types of carbohydrates in our diet: Sugars, Starches, and Cellulose. Simpler than proteins, they are composed of carbon, hydrogen, and oxygen - no nitrogen or sulfur. The basic difference between sugars and starches is the arrangement of the carbon atoms; with starches being simply long chains of sugar units. Cellulose has no nutritional value, but is excellent FIBER.

Since carbohydrates burn much more efficiently than either proteins or fats, they are our most economical source of energy. In fact, they provide about 50% of our energy needs.

By now, most people know that eating refined sugar is extremely unhealthy, generating destructive free radicals during digestion. Sugar also causes rapid aging of the skin, and tooth decay. Refined sugar is right behind animal fats as being among the worst foods for human consumption.

The old misconception about honey being healthier than table (refined) sugar is entirely false. Both table sugar and the sugar in honey are simple sucrose, and are chemically identical to the sucrose in sugar cane. Fructose is the sweetener found in fruits, and

The body can manufacture its own carbohydrates from other natural foods, so there is never a need to be concerned about carbohydrate deficiency, if a natural well-balanced diet is maintained.

It is interesting to note that white flour, polished rice, and white sugar are virtually devoid of nutritional value.

Fiber is a non-nutritive carbohydrate, which is, nevertheless, essential for human health. This health factor, also known as bulk, or roughage, is a form of plant cellulose (a carbohydrate) not digestible by humans.   The common forms in our diet are the bran of cereals, and fruit skins. These forms of fiber help sweep the colon by absorbing water to form bulky, soft stools, and provide an environment for the growth of helpful bacteria for the synthesis of such nutrients as Vitamin K.

An adequate intake of fiber plays a major role in the prevention of diverticular disease, constipation, and colon cancer. **Excessive amounts of fiber can be dangerous**, though, because too much can also sweep out needed nutrients, and aggravate an ulcerous condition.

The best dietary sources of fiber are whole grains breads and cereals, and   fruits and vegetables. Bran and special fiber supplements are unnecessary for most people.

3) Fats: Like carbohydrates, fats are composed of carbon, hydrogen, and oxygen; but with less oxygen. Although fats are essential to good health, an excess of animal fat is among the worst mistakes we can make in our consumption of food (the worst are palm oil and coconut oil).   Fats are indispensable to good health. They are a major source of energy, providing nearly twice as many calories per gram as protein.

As we all well know, fatty foods are among the best tasting of foods. That is because fats, also known as lipids, impart juiciness and flavor to such foods as fatty meats and fried foods. Fatty foods are also major contributors to heart disease, vascular disease, and cancer.

Fats are, however, essential to good health. They contribute to our feeling of "fullness" after meals, because of their slow movement through our digestive tract. Fat insulates our body, and protects our vital organs from physical impact. Fats also transport the fat-soluble vitamins A, D, E, and K, assist the clotting mechanism, and participate in hormone synthesis. Unused fats are stored in the form of fatty acids, and used for energy when needed.

Most people think of fats as: Saturated coming from animal sources; Unsaturated coming from vegetable sources.

These popular descriptions, although generally true, are not accurate. Perhaps the simplest method of describing and explaining the different kinds of fats, or lipids, (there is no really simple way) is as follows: Fats (also known as lipids) are composed of Carbon, Hydrogen, and Oxygen. Fats are essentially chains of Carbon atoms, with Hydrogen atoms (and some Oxygen atoms) attached.

Saturated fats are complete, with no space for additional atoms (as the name suggests). Monounsaturated fat has room for one additional hydrogen atom. Polyunsaturated fat has room for more than one additional hydrogen atom. Hydrogenated fats are fats which were unsaturated, but had the missing hydrogen atoms added to make them saturated fats. The result is to convert such items as vegetable shortenings from a liquid to a solid form.

Cholesterol, also a lipid, is a waxy compound. It is a non-essential nutrient of great significance in the body. Most of the cholesterol found in the body, though, is manufactured by the body itself, in the liver.

The heart disease caused by cholesterol is stimulated by saturated fats serving as the starting material from which cholesterol is manufactured in the body.

Saturated fats raise blood cholesterol levels, and are found primarily in egg yolks, red meat, whole milk, cream, butter, and palm and coconut oils.

Polyunsaturated fats tend to lower blood cholesterol, and are from vegetable sources such as corn, sunflower, soya, and cottonseed oils.

Monounsaturated fats also tend to lower blood cholesterol levels, but to a lesser degree; and come from such sources as olive oil and peanut oil.

The average person consumes 40% to 50% of their diet in fats, and would be wise to reduce this intake to about 30% of their caloric intake. Some methods of doing this are to use leaner cuts of fat-trimmed meat, more use of chicken, fish, veal; and more use of fruits and vegetables. Pork, high fat beef, and lamb are very high in saturated fat, and should be avoided as much as possible.

Fats are also an energy food; and are a concentrated source of energy. Fats have more than twice the number of calories per gram than any other food: about 9 calories per gram.

4) Vitamins: Vitamins might most succinctly be described as the elements which enable the chemical reactions to take place that cause the nourishment of existing cells, and the reproduction of new cells. Each vitamin has its own job to do in the body, and each is essential for health, Long Life, vitality, youthfulness, and attractiveness.

In order to determine your exact vitamin and mineral requirements, some simple blood analyses and practical applications must be made by a doctor and a laboratory.

Generally though, the RDA should be adequate for you, with additional anti-oxidants such as Vitamin E and Beta-Carotene, and Vitamin C. The amounts for you, personally, can only be determined by a Licensed (ask to see the State license) nutritionist who has access to your medical history.

The Known Vitamins Are

Light
Vitamin F
Vitamin A
Vitamin K
Vitamin C (ascorbic acid)
Vitamin P (bioflavonoids)
Vitamin D
Vitamin T
Vitamin E (tocopherol)
Vitamin U

And the B-Complex Vitamins:
Vitamin B1 (Thiamin)
Vitamin B15 (Pangamic Acid)
Vitamin B2 (Riboflavin)
Vitamin B17 (Laetrile)
Vitamin B3 (Niacin)
Biotin
Vitamin B5 (Pantothenic Acid)
Choline
Vitamin B6 (Pyridoxine)
Folic Acid

Vitamin B12 (Cyanocobalamin)
Inositol
Vitamin B13 (Orotic Acid)
PABA (para-aminobenzoic acid)

** **Water-soluble vitamins** are measured in milligrams
    (Mg.)
** **Fat-soluble vitamins** measured in International Units
    (I.U.)

Light

Light, like the good food we eat, is taken into our bodies, and is used in many of our metabolic processes. It is just as vital a nutrient as the vitamins and minerals we consume. Most of the light that we get however, is sadly deficient in the "light nutrition" that we need for health, vitality, attractiveness, and psychological well being.

The complete light nutrition that we require comes only from **Full Spectrum Light**. The sun's light provides the best source of full-spectrum light, which includes light from ultraviolet, through the visual range, into infra-red.

Full-spectrum light reaches the earth at sea level in a band extending from 290 to 3500 "manometers". This entire spectrum of light is vital for the function of all of those chemical reactions within the body that are stimulated by light. When any part of the light spectrum is missing from your light sources, certain body functions required for health, vitality, and attractiveness are not stimulated. Since ordinary artificial light covers only a band from about 375 to 790 manometers, much is lost daily in terms of health maintenance from necessary light stimulation.

No ultraviolet light, so necessary for good health, is provided by these artificial light sources. **Be Aware, Though, That Our Need For Ultra-Violet Light Is Very**

Small, And That <u>All Three Types Are Damaging To Our Life, Health, And Attractiveness</u>: <u>UV-A</u>: Deep penetrating rays. Excess can cause malignant melanoma, the most dangerous form of skin cancer. <u>UV-B</u>: Burns and damages the surface layers of the skin, and causes such skin cancers as basal cell carcinoma, etc. <u>UV-C</u> is blocked by the earth's ozone layer.

<u>Sun lamps</u> such as those used in tanning salons use the longer UV-A rays, which can cause the most dangerous type of skin cancer, malignant melanoma. They don't use the shorter UV-B rays because those are the rays that burn the surface of the skin causing "sunburn".

If you must be in the sun, protect yourself by using a good quality waterproof sunscreen of SPF (Sun Protection Factor) of 15 or greater, that contains benzophenones and cinnamates, which absorb both UVA and UVB light. PABA absorbs <u>only</u> UVB rays, so it prevents "sunburn" of the surface of the skin, but since it does not block UV-A rays, it does <u>not</u> prevent malignant melanoma, the most dangerous form of skin cancer.

The sunscreen should be applied to all parts of the body that are to be exposed, prior to exposure. The most important thing to remember about using sunscreens is to use them frequently and generously. SPF-15 means that 15 hours in the sun with the sunscreen is equal to 1 hour in the sun without it. SPF lotions of greater than 15 do not appear to provide significantly greater protection than does SPF-15.

Fluorescent lighting provides an even more limited spectrum than the ordinary light bulb; and the commonly used "cool-white" provides an even narrower band yet. The cool-white fluorescent tubes have a great insufficiency of ultra-violet radiation, which is vital to our health in moderate quantities; and also have abnormal ratios of red and yellow emissions. This imbalance can cause severe problems to those exposed to it.

Most people know Vitamin D as the "sunshine vitamin". This is because the sun's ultraviolet rays activate dehydrocholesterol in the skin, converting it into Vitamin D.

Vitamin D is essential for the formation and maintenance of good teeth and bones; a stable nervous system; normal heart function; normal blood clotting; and to prevent and fight osteoporosis (brittle bones). Although excessive amounts of ultraviolet rays may be very harmful, moderate amounts are very necessary and healthy for most people.

Insufficient full-spectrum light can cause extreme tension, depression (even suicidal), muscle cramps, anxiety, fatigue, sleeplessness, poor concentration, lack of initiative, low work efficiency; and many other problems resulting from the lack of stimulation by full-spectrum light.

The body requires full-spectrum light in order to utilize many vital nutrients, and to stimulate many of the body's vital functions. For example, the pineal gland in the brain is directly stimulated by light to produce melatonin, which provides for greater stimulation of the nerves by the brain. Deficiencies in this area can influence mood and behavior.

Full-spectrum light is also used in hospitals to prevent and treat *hyperbilirubinemia* in infants; it is used by NASA (National Aeronautics and Space Administration) for space travelers; and the U. S. Navy has used ultraviolet stimulation for submarine personnel.

The "B Complex" Vitamins
These vitamins are grouped together under the term "B Complex", because they generally come from the same foods, and interact closely with one another.

The B Vitamins are active in providing energy by converting carbohydrates into glucose, which the body "burns" for energy. They are vital in the metabolism of fats and protein; and may be the single most important factor for normal functioning of the nervous system, and the health of the nerves. They are essential for maintenance of muscle tone in the gastrointestinal tract, and for the health of skin, hair, eyes, mouth, and liver.

All of the B Vitamins, except B17, are found in brewer's yeast, liver, or whole grain cereals and breads; with brewer's yeast being the richest natural source.

Most preparations of individual B vitamins are synthetic; or at least no longer in their natural form. These synthetic B vitamins are used primarily to overcome severe deficiencies.

Since the B vitamins exert many different effects upon each other; and since excesses and insufficiencies may be harmful, it is important that all of the B Complex vitamins be taken at the same time, in their natural balance; such as they appear in brewer's yeast for example.

B Complex vitamins are not stored in the body, so they must be taken regularly. **They are destroyed by the consumption of sugar and alcohol.**

The B Complex vitamins are so sparsely provided by the national diet, that almost everyone lacks some of them. If a person is tired, irritable, nervous, depressed, lacking in self-confidence, or even suicidal; suspect a B vitamin deficiency.

In addition, gray hair, falling hair, baldness, acne, and many other skin problems are caused by a lack of B vitamins, as is poor appetite, insomnia, neuritis, anemia, constipation, and a high cholesterol level.

Almost all of the B Complex vitamins are found in yeast, which is the first item you may want to consider adding to your diet. This addition to your diet though, should consist of at least 50% brewer's yeast, and the balance can be torula yeast, which is much richer in the B vitamins; but seems to lack an as yet unidentified growth factor, which is present in brewer's yeast. Brewer's yeast is also called "primary" yeast. Again, water-soluble vitamins are measured in milligrams (Mg.), Fat soluble vitamins are measured in International Units (I.U.).

The B Complex Vitamins Are:

B1 (Thiamin)   B15 (Pangamic Acid)
B2 (Riboflavin)   B17 (Laetrile)
B3 (Niacin)   Biotin
B5 (Pantothenic Acid)   Choline
B6 (Pyridoxine)   Folic Acid
B12 (Cyanocobalamin)   Inositol
B13 (Orotic Acid)
PABA (Para-Aminobenzoic Acid)

5) Minerals: Minerals are needed daily and, along with Vitamins, are sometimes called "micronutrients". They are inorganic elements which help to form tissues and other body chemicals. They help to regulate the pH (acid-base) balance of the body and fluid levels, and assist in muscle contraction and nerve transmission.

Minerals are constituents of all tissues and internal fluids, including the bones, teeth, soft tissue, muscle, blood, and nerve cells. They are important factors in all physiological processes, strengthening skeletal structures, and preserving the vigor of the heart and brain, as well as all muscle and nerve systems. Minerals are also important in the production of hormones.

Physical and emotional stress causes a strain on the body's supply of minerals. A mineral deficiency often results in illness, which may be checked by the addition of the missing mineral to the diet.

Minerals not listed here are either not known to be of benefit to the human body, or are toxic (poisonous).

The following minerals are essential in human nutrition. They are vital to mental and physical well-being.:

Calcium	Manganese
Chlorine	Molybdenum
Chromium	Phosphorous
Cobalt	**Potassium**
Copper	Selenium
Fluorine	Sodium
Iodine	Sulfur
Iron	Vanadium
Magnesium	Zinc

And the Essential Trace Minerals, whose role in human nutrition is unknown:

Boron, Lithium, Silicon, Strontium, Tin, and Tritium.

Water And Air

...are the body's most urgently needed nutrients, so a brief explanation is included here, showing how to utilize them best.

Water

Water is by far the most essential of all minerals. It is used in every single process in the body, and no body function can be performed or sustained without sufficient quantities of water.

Tap water (from surface water) may contain pollutants from the air, or from rainwater runoff into the waterways, causing fertilizer or insecticide residue. Chemicals added to tap water to kill bacteria may themselves contain small amounts of poisonous or carcinogenic (cancer-producing) substances.

Well water has a much less uniform mineral content than surface water, but depending on the area, well water can range from nearly no minerals, to excessive amounts. It may also contain "inorganic" minerals which cannot be assimilated by the body.

Boiling water for purity is not recommended. Although all bacteria is killed, the pure water all goes up in steam, and the remaining water may contain unhealthy concentrated amounts of heavy metals or nitrates.

The only "pure" water there is, (100% pure hydrogen and oxygen) is water in fruits and vegetables, and "distilled" water. This pure water, although the best water to consume, has no minerals, so the mineral requirements must be met through mineral-rich foods, or by supplements.

The average adult maintains about 45 quarts of water in the body. They lose through excretion (including perspiration) about 3 quarts per day, depending on activity level and environment (this can range from less than 1 quart, to 10 quarts per day in a very hot climate).

The daily intake of water by drinking water and various liquids, and by consuming water contained in foods, should be sufficient to maintain the body's required water level. Large deficiencies of water should be corrected as soon as possible.

The old story of not drinking liquids while exercising is incorrect. Small amounts of liquid should be consumed throughout the exercise period, as needed.

Air

Sufficient oxygen is the most urgent human need, not just for good health and attractiveness but for life itself. We take an average of about 16 breaths per minute, every day of our lives. Even the strongest and healthiest of us could not stay alive more than a few minutes without taking a breath of air containing oxygen.

Breathing in is called "inspiration", and breathing out is called "expiration". The total air the lungs can hold is 3 to 5 quarts, depending on the individual's capacity. This total amount is called "vital capacity". The air that passes in and out during ordinary breathing is "tidal air", and is about 500 cc (cubic centimeters) of air.

After a normal expiration, you can forcibly breathe in about 3,000 cc of air. This air is called "complemental air". After a normal expiration, you can force out about another 1,000 cc of air. This air is called "supplemental air".

No matter how hard you blow out, there always remains in the lungs about 1,000 to 1,500 cc of air. This is called "residual air".

Thus, during ordinary breathing we use only about one-eighth of our lung capacity, so a large part of our lungs don't receive fresh air with each breath. This is the primary reason that occasional deep breathing is so vital. Air does not circulate within the lungs themselves. Stale air remains in the unused portion of the lungs until a deep enough breath is taken to replace it. Insufficient oxygen creates a variety of health problems such as impaired brain functioning and memory, reduced nerve sensations, and loss of brain cells.

Breathing should be deep and regular, with the stomach protruding on the intake of breath. Conversely, hyperventilating is also unhealthy because it results in low CO_2 levels. In addition to being a waste product of oxygen metabolism, CO_2 aids in maintaining our pH balance. Low CO_2 levels constrict the blood vessels and can contribute to stroke, migraine headache, cancer, epilepsy, and angina pectoris.

Filling the lungs more completely expands and stimulates them, bringing fresh air and fresh circulation into all areas of the lungs. It is not commonly known that the lungs themselves do not actively expand and contract in the breathing process. This is done by the movement of the diaphragm (the large, dome-shaped muscle which separates the abdomen from the chest), and by the chest muscles - especially the small muscles attached to the ribs.

The best method of sustaining a healthy respiratory system is to perform daily exercise which causes us to breathe very deeply for at least 10 minutes, in a reasonably clean air area (not a busy street).

Essential Trace Minerals
Lithium, Boron, Strontium, Silicon, Tin, and Tritium are essential trace minerals which the body needs, but whose role in human nutrition is not yet known. A nutrition program that provides sufficient of the other essential minerals should satisfy the need for these trace minerals.

Carl Bourhenne, MA
Gerontologist

Carl Bourhenne's

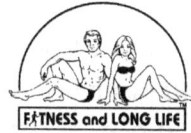

FITNESS and LONG LIFE

How To Live
The Longest Life Possible

Stress Control

Occupation, Rest and Relaxation

The importance **STRESS** of Rest and Relaxation for Long Life is so profound that expressing its value adequately requires great effort. Indeed, understanding the importance of Rest and Relaxation for a healthy long life takes a deep understanding of the devastating enemy which we call "stress".

The following presentation on stress is intended to be an important lead-in to the section on Rest and Relaxation.

Stress

Excessive stress can cause any degree of harm to people, from mild discomfort, to disease and crippling, and even death. The word "stress", though, is commonly used in two different ways, and this can be confusing.

1. It is sometimes used to denote **a cause of stress (stressor),**

2. and at other times it is used to denote **the result of the stressor inside the person under stress (stress, itself).** **To avoid confusion this section will use the two words <u>stressor</u>, and <u>stress</u>, as follows:**

1. The word "**<u>stressor</u>**" will refer to anything that **TENDS** to produce a stressful response.

2. The word "**<u>stress</u>**" will refer to **A Person's <u>Internal Response</u> To A "Stressor". This is something that a person does, and is controllable...it is <u>NOT</u> AN UNCONTROLLABLE RESPONSE.**

Knowledge in the subject of stress as a health factor was greatly advanced by the well-known stress researcher Hans Selye, a physiologist at the University of Montreal. Selye showed that stressors can come from **outside** of us, or from **inside** of us (our imagination, etc.). He also showed that a person's response to stress can have both mental and physical components, and that the mental and physical reactions can even interact with each other.

Selye showed that stress is a demand on us to adapt - either to a negative event such as an argument - or to a positive event such as love-making; so stress is not all bad. He showed too that extreme positive stress can be harmful, just as can extreme negative stress.

So, it is not the fact of a stressful event that is harmful to us, or even whether it is a positive (a new job) or a negative event; but, rather **<u>the harm comes when the stress is extreme or prolonged</u>**.

The determination of whether or not stress is harmful to us re lates to **the three stages of stress**, as described by Selye.

The Three Stages Of Stress

1) Alarm   2) Resistance   3) Exhaustion

In **the first stage of stress, the Alarm stage**, the body adapts to the stressor by activating the autonomic nervous system and the endocrine system.   Adrenaline, noradrenaline, and corticosteroids are poured into the bloodstream.   The heart rate and blood pressure are increased, as are the amount of oxygen, glucose, cholesterol, and some free fatty acids in the blood. The basal metabolic rate is raised, blood is shifted from the gastrointestinal tract toward the head and extremities, the number of one type of white blood cell (eosinophils) is decreased in the blood, and the brain's electrical activity is altered. We might not even notice these changes, depending on the severity of the stressor and on our awareness of our responses. At first we are upset and alarmed by these stressors, but we adapt and get used to them.

In **the second stage of stress, the Resistance stage**, we begin to use all of the forces which we marshaled during the Alarm stage, to resist the stressor. How long this goes on depends on the type and intensity of the stressor. Obviously, the longer it goes on, the more we are depleting and taxing the abilities, energies, and resources we activated during the Alarm stage.

If the stressor continues until we exhaust the abilities, energies, and resources activated in the Alarm stage and used up in the Resistance stage then,

The third stage of stress, the Exhaustion stage, sets in. The body's adaptation resources are used up and the person begins to suffer damage, and eventually dies, if the stressor is severe enough and continues long enough.

Autopsies on Selye's experimental rats who died of stress, showed the ravages of stress taken to the Exhaustion stage:

Enlarged adrenal glands, atrophied lymph nodes and thymus glands, and gastrointestinal ulcers.

We might not be aware of the harmful effects of situations to which we think we have become accustomed, such as strenuous labor in extreme heat or cold, a frustrating romantic relationship, eyesight irritants, or relational conflicts; but repeated or continual exposure to stressors may be doing us more harm than we know.

We may become emotionally accustomed to the stressor, but the physical component will continue, breaking down the heart, blood vessels, hormones in the blood, nervous system functioning, and other organs and systems. In time, the final effect can be death from the accumulated damage.

In fact, stress has been associated by researchers with a wide variety of diseases, both mental and physical. Research has shown decidedly that stress can be a contributing cause of heart attacks, cancer, ulcers, diabetes, leukemia, infections, and even sudden death.

People experiencing stress have also been shown to have more accidents, athletic injuries, display neurotic symptoms, attempt suicide, and be hospitalized for depression and schizophrenia.

Stressors generate different levels of stress response, and each person responds to stressors in his or her own way and in varying degrees of stress reaction.

What might TEND to stimulate an extremely stressful response in one person might be NO STRESS AT ALL for another person.

One of the reasons for the different effect which a given stressor can have on different people is that **people perceive**

events in different ways. One employee might see a call from the boss as a threat of criticism, and another employee might see it as an opportunity to shine. Another reason for the different effect of a stressor on different people is the degree of impact the stressor might have. If a family man is turned down for a raise, the impact on his lifestyle can be significant, but a single man might not be as effected.

It is important to be aware of the fact that, since a stressor can be anything that calls on us to make any adaptation of any kind, stressors can be negative or positive events.

Damage only occurs when the demand and response of adaptation continues into the Exhaustion stage.

Thus, losing one's job can be a stressful event, but so can getting married and going on vacation, because they all call for some sort of adaptation, or adjustment.

If we adapt to these events in a smooth and timely way, we might suffer no harmful effects of stress. But if we do not adapt smoothly and in a timely way to such an event, we might suffer some degree of damage as a result of having to contend with the adaptation into Exhaustion.

Such major changes in people's lives as those mentioned - changes for better or for worse - are among the most significant stressors in regard to a healthy Long Life.

Two of the best known researchers who have tried to measure the stressful effects of various life changes on people are Dr. Thomas H. Holmes of the University of Washington, Seattle, and Dr. Richard H. Rahe of the San Diego Naval Health Research Center. They listed 43 typical life events, and after some research they assigned a stress value to each life event.

They call it The Social Readjustment Rating Scale, with each event having a rating in Life Change Units (LCU's) of 1 to 100, with 100 being the most stressful.

The items range from minor violations of the law = 11 LCU's, and vacation = 13 LCU's, through trouble with the boss = 23 LCU's and retirement = 45 LCU's, to divorce = 73 LCU's, and death of a spouse = 100 LCU's (the highest score).

Another major type of stressor is environmental stressors. Air pollution, excessive noise, extreme heat or cold, inadequate light, excessive sunlight, etc., can all have a negative impact on us.

So, now that we are aware of the possible dangers of stress, what do we do to protect our health and promote our own Long Life in view of these dangers?

The first approach is to <u>Avoid Unnecessary Stressors</u>. Control the amount and quality of time you spend with people who tend to generate a stressful response which you have great difficulty managing - family and friends as well as co-workers and acquaintances. Avoid extremes such as overeating, drinking too much, lack of sleep, and overwork. Don't procrastinate. Identify what you, yourself consider to be your own responsibilities, and perform them well. You might consider changing jobs - either for a different type of work, or for different people to work with.

Remember though, **not all stress is harmful, and some stress is necessary** for you to respond to the challenges of personal growth and daily living requirements. Some degree of concern, and even fear are not only normal, but necessary for dealing with stressful events.

In general, if your response to a stressor leaves you feeling happy and healthy, it is probably beneficial, and not one which will result in exhaustion of your internal resources. If you are unsure of whether you need to make a change to relieve stress, you may want to speak with someone you can trust.

Here are some guidelines for handling pressure to avoid stress, from the U.S. Department of Health, Education, and Welfare's National Institute of Mental Health:

Pressure is a normal part of everyday life. If you know how to deal with it, you can actually spur creativity, productivity, and healthy relationships with others. If you let it get out of hand, it can become a problem.

If you have trouble handling pressure and using it constructively, here are some tips:

How You Can Handle Pressure

1. Confide in someone you can trust. Talking about a problem often helps to reduce tension, and another person can offer suggestions from his or her perspective.
2. If you're afraid of something, admit it to yourself. It's nothing to be ashamed of. Everyone has been in the same boat at one time or another.
3. Don't try to escape a problem with lines like "I'll snap out of it", or "It's them, not me."
   You won't convince anyone - least of all yourself.
4. Don't take out your problems on your friends, family, or co-workers. It doesn't make you feel any better, and it makes them miserable too.
5. If you're quarreling with someone, remember that it's just possible that you could be wrong. If you yield some ground, others will.
6. Competition induces pressure because other people become threats to you. Try cooperation instead - It's

contagious! You may make life easier for several people, including yourself.

7. Don't always stick with a problem until you solve it. You may do better to let it lie and to relax or take on another task. When you return to your problem, you may find you approach it from a new and refreshed viewpoint.

8. Take your mind off your problems by doing something for someone else.

9. Take time out for fun - a baseball game, a movie, or a long walk. Relaxation absorbs pressure like a sponge, so be sure to build it into your schedule.

In addition to these methods of handling pressure, there are some well-established methods for controlling our responses to stressors:

1) We can reduce the intensity of our psychological reactions to stressors, and

2) We can try looking at stressors from different points of view in order to see them in better perspective.

We can also reduce our physical response to stressors by relaxing the muscles which may have tensed, such as the neck, shoulder, chest, stomach, and extremity muscles; and we can induce normal deep breathing if it has tensed up.

Other commonly practiced techniques may require, or may best be guided by professionals:

Physical Relaxation: A technique for relaxing all of the muscles in an organized fashion is used by athletes in preparation for competition. This method calls for lying flat on your back and progressively relaxing every muscle in the body, beginning at the top of the head and moving down to the toes. One approach is to tense each muscle first, then relax it. The end feeling is that the bones are lying directly on the mat or mattress.

Mental Relaxation can be a separate method, or a part of this method. Simply try to relax the mind until it seems to contain non-specific thoughts.

Meditation is a technique in which one assumes a very relaxed position, and casually thinks only pleasant thoughts, or concentrates on one certain sound or phrase. **Transcendental Meditation**, commonly called **TM**, may be learned from books, classes, or in practicing groups.

Several approaches are taken by various leaders and groups; but perhaps the best approach for purposes of stress-reduction may be that which trains the individual to control physiological responses. Muscle tension, oxygen consumption, and even pulse rate and blood pressure can be controlled with practice.

Yoga, and some of the martial arts use some of their techniques as stress control methods.

Biofeedback: This technique does not work for everyone, and can be expensive and time-consuming. The person learning control is hooked up to electronic instruments which may monitor brain waves, pulse rate, respiration, muscle contraction, and perspiration.

The person receives audio or/and visual signals from the instruments, and thus learns to control such functions as muscle tension, blood pressure, blood vessel constriction, pulse rate, and brain waves.

Exercise: The results of exercise, especially strenuous exercise include enlisting muscles, arterioles, and other body systems which may be involved in an ongoing tense, or stressful response. This forces the release of the tense, or stressed condition. Exercise may also release psychological tension, and even burn off stress hormones.

Exercise may be the best method of all to eliminate a stressful condition because, in addition to releasing both mental and physical stress, it circulates nutrients and oxygen to the stressed areas.

Drugs: Tranquilizers and mild sedatives can be prescribed by doctors, but the possibility of dependency and side effects make them less attractive than learning the independent methods described above.

A glass of wine each day has been touted in some of the longevity literature as contributive to long life because of the stress-reducing reaction, but the harmful effects of alcohol on the system make this a questionable way to reduce stress.

Since the objective of this book, **How To Live The Longest Life Possible,** is to present lifestyle habits as contributors to a healthy Long Life, this section discussing general lifestyle attitudes as they relate to stress has been saved for last, in order that it might be best remembered.

Control of daily lifestyle habits is, indeed, the most important and most effective way to a stress - controlled Long Life. To arrange one's life into a harmonious, smooth-flowing series of events in which one is in tune with one's self, with one's family, friends, co-workers, and acquaintances, and with one's material world (that is, that one's material and financial needs are met), is to arrange for an excessively stress-free existence.

However, to be unfulfilled is itself a highly stressful condition; so, we do want to fulfill ourselves and meet our goals. We want to do so, though, in a way that promotes congeniality, without creating conflict within ourselves or in the world around us.

That is stress, that is what it can do to us, and those are some important approaches to dealing with and alleviating stress. Perhaps as important though is the long life recommendation, that we all set aside some time each day, each week, each month, and each year for rest and relaxation; because that may be one of the best ways to release stress reactions begun recently. The objective of this rest and relaxation, from a health and long life point of view, is to dissolve stress which has begun, before it reaches stage 3 - the devastating **Exhaustion** stage of stress described above.

The act of setting aside time for rest and relaxation suggests a decision to spend such time involved in the form of rest and relaxation decided upon, essentially to the exclusion of other involvements. This decision, and involvement in the planned rest and relaxation, should result in release of all accumulated stresses - or may with practice.

One of the most effective and beneficial forms of rest and relaxation is a mid-day nap, which can add many years of healthy long life.

So, be aware that **stress is one of the worst things that can happen to a human being. Stress causes more deaths each year than smoking, overweight, and lack of exercise, Combined.** Stress also causes rapid aging, and the appearance of aging early and fast.

Stress Causes Damage In Three Primary Ways:

1) The muscle tension of stress closes circulation to various parts of the body, including vital organs, for extended periods of time. This denies nutrition and oxygen from being distributed via the blood supply. The result is the death of body cells, and of organs.

2) Stress causes mass adverse chemical reactions throughout the body, upsetting bio-chemical functions necessary for the continuance of life, health, and attractiveness. Research is presently being conducted which may show that the here-to-fore unknown cause of the adherence of plaque to arterial walls, causing coronary occlusion and heart damage, may be caused by the adverse chemical reactions of the body to stress

3) Stress is also known to instantly drain the body of vital nutrients, such as C, and the B Complex vitamins. The body then ages rapidly until they are replaced.

The most visible results of stress are deep wrinkles and lines in the face and neck, puffiness of the face - especially around the eyes, with bagging under the eyes.

Some of **the immediate results of stress** are, tightness in the chest, shortness of breath, lack of stamina, and impatience.

Some of **the common reactions to stress** are anger, the urge for heavy smoking, excessive eating - especially of sweets, and heavy drinking. Also, we do not function well under stress. That is why the hard-and-fast driving executive is now known to be less successful than his more relaxed, thoughtful, pleasant, counterpart, for whom people are more willing to work with enthusiasm.

Stress can actually become a bad habit one forms as a reaction to intense situations in which we may or may not feel competent. These situations may be personal, social, business, or even recreational.

Occupation

Oddly enough, it is the two occupational extremes: Highest level jobs, in which you have no boss, and Jobs consisting of hard physical labor that hold the promise of longest life.

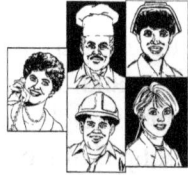

The single exception to this is the medical profession, where the risks of exposure to germs, infection, diseases, and X-rays outweigh the advantages of self-employment. A medical doctor can add significantly (3 to 13 years) to his or her life expectancy by taking extreme caution against infection, and by avoiding frequent contact with X-ray equipment and procedures.

So, if you are not already in one of those two categories, you can add several (10 to 13) years to your life by:
1) Become the top executive of another company.
2) Own your own business.
3) Have a job doing hard physical labor.

A housewife in a well-to-do home is also in the better occupation category for health and long life.

No matter what kind of work you choose to do, though, some interesting information can help you to prevent the stress of your job from damaging your health and appearance, or from shortening your life.

In general, for instance, the more intense and regimented your work is, the less time you should spend doing it. If you work on a production line doing the same thing over and over, with a time limit for each task, you are under much more strain than a person who is not forced to follow a rigid schedule. So, a person in a highly regimented job should work at least 2 hours per week less than the person who works on a loose schedule.

The solution, however, to working stress free, especially on a highly regimented job, is to make it a point, every hour, to stand up, raise the arms over the head for a few moments and stretch; then relax the neck, shoulders, chest, and take a couple of slow, deep breaths.

Then, in the middle of the work day, do a few exercises that will vigorously move and stretch most of the body muscles, getting the arms up over the head, causing you to breathe fast.

For the final, ideal touch, a nap at midday can add many years of healthy long life, youthful and attractive, to your life.

Carl Bourhenne, MA
Gerontologist

Carl Bourhenne's

FITNESS and LONG LIFE

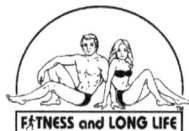

How To Live
The Longest Life Possible

Stay Active
Recreation, Community, Work

The concept of "use it or lose it" in regard to health and long life is probably no new rule to you. In fact, it is probably one of the most used terms in discussions of how to stay healthy over time.

The directive to stay active through work, recreation, and community activities addresses a wide range of human abilities most people want to keep. The process of work involves the use of mind, emotions, and to varying degrees the body; as do recreation and community activities.

Recreation

In addition to the relaxation value of recreation, most recreational activities involve one or more basic health-promoting activities. These activities, besides using and thus keeping many faculties, also help to maintain various aspects of our health. For instance, many sports and games have exercise value. Many forms of recreation provide exceptional mental stimulation; and most involve some social interaction.

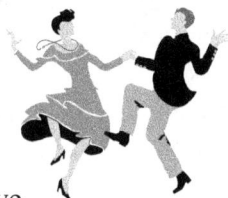

All of the faculties used are maintained by the fact of their healthy use.

Community Activities

In the three areas of the world where large percentages of the populations live to advanced ages healthy and active,

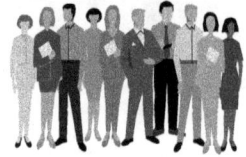

1. **The Abkhasians in the Caucasus Mountains of Soviet Georgia.** (The most famous)
2. **The Vilcabambans in the Ecuadorian Andes.**
3. **The Hunzas in the Karakorum Mountains of Kashmir in West Pakistan's Himalayas.**

It was shown that involvement in community activities is the norm. There is no retirement from involvement in the community. Each of the inhabitants, regardless of age, has a role to play in community affairs and activities, and thus maintains a sense of social worth.

It is not only the personal faculties that are maintained; but the joy of life and the excitement of participation, as well.

Work

Depending on the type of work one prefers, the use of such faculties as observation, memory, learning, judgment, decision-making, creativity, and other abilities are used. Most work situations also involve social interactions to some extent; so the many facets of social relations are stimulated, and thus maintained.

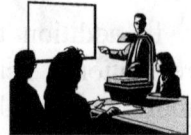

Work also provides the much needed feeling of being valuable.

Carl Bourhenne's

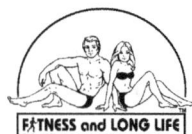

How To Live
The Longest Life Possible

Social Activity

Sexuality, Friends, Family

Stay **Involved With Family And Friends.** As human beings we are social animals. We do not seem able to exist in isolation as some other organisms do. We need to develop some form of society and obtain the company and support of other human beings. We need others even to provide the necessities of life such as food, clothing, housing, and security against our enemies. Ever since the beginning of man we have formed societies; and everywhere on earth where human beings are, they have banded together and formed societies of some kind.

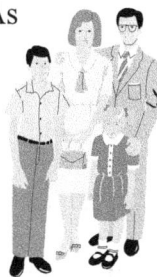

Several research results show that we need some kind of love or attention to be healthy, emotionally. In fact, the lack of love and human companionship contribute to serious disease, and even to death. The renowned Abraham Maslow includes the need for affection as one of our basic needs, along with food, water, security, and self esteem.

One of the many reasons for staying involved with family and friends is to help fill their needs, especially those of our parents. As they age, their friends tend to become fewer and fewer, by attrition; so they need us more and more to fill their needs for love and affection.

For ourselves as well, our family and friends provide the largest share of our love and affection. We have basic ties with our family, and special memories of sharing and growth. Our friends have, for the most part, been chosen because we perceive them to be like ourselves, because they are familiar to us; because they like us, because they are good at what they do; and because we find them attractive. We have met many people in the process of establishing friendships with these few people, and we would do ourselves well to stay in touch with these valuable friends who, with our families, provide our vital needs for love and affection.

We are all aware that an active social life is not only one of the most fun, fulfilling, pleasurable, satisfying, and informative aspects of living; but, in addition, many major research programs completed in the last few years on the subject of aging (including the Russians, who are among the most prodigious researchers on health, long life, and the aging process), listed as one of the most important conclusions that an active social life is an absolute must for a healthy, long life - especially later in life.

In fact, a major conclusion listed is that the "lone wolf" tends to live the shortest life span and be less healthy, physically and emotionally.

It is ill advised to be a "lone wolf", and recent studies show that social involvement should include:
1) Have several close friends whom you see regularly, get along with them, and develop common interests with

them.

2) Participate regularly in group social activities.
3) Fulfill an important role in your community in some way that makes you feel an important part.

4) **Don't hold grudges!** This is one of the most important mental attitudes displayed by each of the societies where people live the longest lives. They all got along well with one another, they readily forgive and forget all transgressions, and there were never any ill feelings. No matter what happens, they hold no grudges.

Much of the research completed to date shows that married people tend to live longer and be healthier than their single counterparts. This may, however, prove to have been due, at least in part, to the pressure of the times. Future research will clarify this point further. These studies do show clearly that people who had experienced divorces - especially several - lived much shorter lives than those who remained married to their first spouse.

More recent trends have been toward a broader acceptance of the single status. Living single, and living with and separating from several partners over a period of time does not involve the same amount of stress that it once did. Social attitudes, financial prosperity, automation, and ease of meeting new people nave significantly lessened the stress involved in separation from a domestic situation.

Sexuality

Although sexual activity is not one of the basic requirements for the immediate continuation of life itself, some of the most dramatic research results have emerged from the studies performed on the healthy aspects of regularly sexual activity. The difference between people who had regular sexual activity and those who did not, or who were celibate, leads us to wonder if sexual activity is not more important than was formerly believed.

Physical appearance and health of both men and women was of significantly higher quality as life progressed.

It is now clear that regular sexual activity may prevent many types of illness and disease, because it avoids or releases stress.

In addition, research into the inner workings of the body shows that orgasm in both men and women results in the release into the body of many beneficial chemicals.

Two major research centers have independently documented what is now commonly termed the **"Late In Life Cause Of Aging"**.

These independent studies each showed that **when sexual activity ceased in older people, they experienced a more rapid decline of their health**.

The post-mortem physical examinations given to both test groups led to the conclusion that **the continuation of sexual activity, especially in later life, contributes greatly not only to health, but also to their physical youthfulness**.

Older people have always been active, sexually, even into their 90's and 100, and beyond.

They have traditionally not talked about it so as not to shock their children and grandchildren. **But older people have always been quite active, sexually**.

The truth is that people can be sexually active as long as they are alive and reasonably healthy.

And, contrary to popular opinion, the sex drive does not even diminish all that much, and then only gradually.

If someone experiences a dramatic decline in sex drive, they should seek help. And adequate help is readily available.

Masturbation is a natural and healthy activity for both men and women. It has been said that 98% of all men masturbate and the other 2% are liars. While that might be an overstatement of reality, it seems to represent what is natural.

For both women and men to increase the intensity of their orgasm, and for men to regain the ability for orgasm, practice the "KEGEL" Exercise: act as though you are trying to keep from peeing. Google it for more.

In the event that the woman has been sexually abstinent for a period of 3 to 5 years or more, the use of K-Y Jelly or some other non-alcoholic, non-petroleum lubricant designed for compatibility with the chemistry of the vagina may adequately alleviate discomfort in sexual intercourse.

It is especially important for women to maintain their sexual health when they do not have a partner, because the vagina loses both its elasticity and its ability to lubricate if it is neglected for up to about a five years.

For this reason it is important for a woman to utilize object insertion during masturbation in order for the vagina to maintain its elasticity and its ability to lubricate. Otherwise if she resumes sexual activity after a long period of complete sexual abstinence, intercourse could be very painful.

The alternatives to these effects are activity, especially continued regular sexual activity, exercise, good nutrition, and good health habits.

Petroleum products such as baby oil and Vaseline must never be put in or on the vagina, as they will upset the pH balance of the vagina, making it susceptible to yeast infections and other problems.

The old adage that **an exercise program can rejuvenate the sex drive** is true. If you don't believe it, I recommend that you try it. It's only fair to warn your mate though. Otherwise they might wonder what suddenly got into you.

Any modern discussion on sexuality must address the subject of AIDS (Acquired Immune Deficiency Syndrome). Not only must the sexually active person today take steps to protect himself and herself from the threat of STD's (Sexually Transmitted Diseases, formerly known as VD - Venereal Disease), but today they must protect themselves against AIDS, a life threatening disease transmitted by sexual intercourse, including anal intercourse, and by the exchange of body fluids including the swallowing of vaginal fluids or semen. So the newly popular rhyme: **"A Tisket, A Tasket, A Condom Or A Casket"** is one worth remembering at that special time when one would least like to think of it.

Another important notion from the social aspect of living for health, youthfulness, and attractiveness, is to **maintain "Emotional Stability"**.

Emotional stability means, in this context, maintaining a positive attitude always, while avoiding over-reacting to adverse conditions and adverse social experiences. It is very stressful to allow an extreme negative reaction to outside, or even to inner adverse situations.

Actually, if we always look at the other person's viewpoint, we may well understand why they did what they did, and not over-react.

A man once said, "If I wanted to make my worst enemy miserable, I'd make him hate someone". And that's how it works. Love and Liking are contributors to our health, youthfulness, and long life; but dislike of others is destructive. And, if there is someone we don't enjoy being around, we can simply stay away from them. Remember, **the opposite of love is not hate; it is indifference**.

In summary, **don't be a "lone wolf"**. Develop several close friends (even though no one is perfect, neither are you; and we all need social interactions).

Be a valuable part of your community, participate in group social activities, enjoy a sex life that is normal for you, maintain emotional stability, and **Never Hold A Grudge -- It will shorten YOUR life!**

Follow these precepts and you can be healthier longer, and stay more youthful and more attractive.

Carl Bourhenne, MA
Gerontologist

Carl Bourhenne's

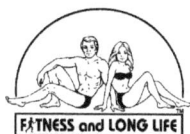

How To Live
The Longest Life Possible

Sleep

Even in today's world of modern research with its abundant fruit of explanations and answers, there is as yet no agreement on why we sleep, or even what triggers sleep. As one researcher, W.C. Dement stated: "Never in the history of biological research has so much been known about something from a descriptive point of view with so little known at the same time about its function". Even so, research on Long Life clearly demonstrates that getting enough sleep is necessary for living a long, healthy life.

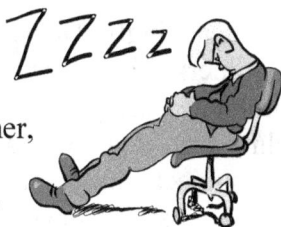

It is possible though, that no damage occurs from losing sleep - even large amounts - and then making it up. Our friend Dement watched while 17 year old Randy Gardner surpassed the Guinness world record for staying awake in 1965, by remaining awake for 11 consecutive days. Although there was increasing sleepiness, there were no signs of psychotic behavior, paranoia, or personality change. It took him only 14 hours and 40 minutes of sleep to awaken fully refreshed, and his second night's sleep was only 8 hours. Follow-up studies on Randy Gardner showed no long-term problems in sleep, no emotional upsets, and no personality changes.

Even though we would assume that without sleep the body would deteriorate in some important physical or biochemical way, research shows otherwise. After 2 days you might feel fatigued, depressed, lethargic, hostile, and less happy; experience a decline in the ability to concentrate or do motor, visual, or perceptual tasks; and may experience a ravenous appetite. After 5 days there might be hallucinations such as seeing a gorilla. Even after these prolonged periods of sleeplessness, though, there may be no remarkable changes in heart rate, blood pressure, perspiration, or body temperature. In certain individuals psychotic behavior may occur; but this is related to personality.

Interestingly, Dement concluded after his observations of Gardner: "The crucial factor in surmounting the effects of prolonged sleep loss is probably physical fitness. There is almost no degree of sleepiness that cannot be overcome if the subject engages in vigorous exercise. As the vigil wears on, almost continuous muscular activity is necessary to forestall overwhelming sleepiness. Many individuals simply would not be able to maintain this amount of activity, and would therefore appear to succumb to the debilitating effects of sleep loss."

So, while losing sleep and then making it up does not appear to cause physical, psychological, or biochemical damage, getting enough sleep generally, does appear to be a major factor in promoting Long Life.

How much sleep do we need, though? Why do you need 8 hours every night, and our neighbor only 6 hours; or vice versa? Vast amounts of research have been performed attempting to determine the ideal amount of sleep. The answer is that each person has their own ideal amount of sleep; and that it is probably inherited, at least partly. The research shows that 92% of people need between 6 1/2 and 9 1/2 hours of sleep per night (24 hour period); with the other 8% requiring either more, or less in varying amounts. There are records of people who functioned normally on 3 hours sleep per night, and it is not known if their brain chemistry was different from others'.

There are no observable personality differences among people based on their sleep requirement. There are no differences in intelligence; nor is there a difference in the amounts of sleep needed between men and women, generally. Those who sleep erratically and often miss the greater part of a night's sleep have the shortest life spans; and those who habitually sleep more than nine hours per night have the second-shortest life span.

The sleep requirement for an individual may be altered slightly, but only with great effort. After reducing sleep time from 8 to 5 hours by going to bed later and getting up at the same time, some subjects experienced extreme difficulty in getting up in the morning, fatigue, less vigor, difficulty in concentrating, and felt less friendly and happy. Unwanted mood changes discouraged them from going below 5 hours; but, when these subjects went back to a schedule of their choosing, most of them were found to sleep 1 to 2 hours less than before the study began. So, if you sleep 8 hours, you might, with great effort and probably much discomfort, be able to reduce your sleeping time to 7, or possibly 6 hours; but probably not less.

Does it make a difference what time of the day we sleep? What is this "jet-lag" business? Biological responses that have a 24 hour cycle are called circadian rhythms. Circadian means "about a day". Although you probably inherited your own circadian rhythm, you may be able to modify your sleep rhythm somewhat. Your circadian rhythms are probably controlled by chemical secretions from various areas in the brain. You would probably function on this cycle and sleep the same number of hours whether you were living in a cave, in an area of constant light, or in a hospital bed. Disabled people who lie in bed all day sleep about the same as active persons. Although most people are awake for about 16 hours each day and sleep for about 8 hours, there is no one answer to why you go to sleep or stay awake. The specific trigger is thought to be one of the chemicals involved in sleep; but if your circadian rhythm is interrupted you may be unable to go to sleep even though very fatigued. Most of us have experienced feeling too fatigued to sleep; but it is usually the deviation from our cycle that inhibits sleep.

Past research concentrated on 5 stages of sleep; but many theories regarding the various stages were disproved, and one recent scientist, Laverne Johnson, concluded that you can function normally after missing some of the stages.

Johnson suggested lumping the five sleep stages into two sleep states:
1. Quiet Sleep **(QS)** - also referred to as Non-Rapid Eye Movement sleeps (NREM).
2. Active Sleep **(AS)** - also referred to as Rapid Eye Movement sleeps (REM).

Let's use the newer terms **QS (Quiet Sleep)**, and **AS (Active Sleep)** to denote these two sleep states.

The first sleep state, **Quiet Sleep (QS)**, usually begins just after falling asleep, and lasts for 40 to 80 minutes. It is generally assumed, though not proven, that one function of **QS** is to help us recover from the fatigue of the day. So **QS** helps us to restore our energy for the coming day. We do dream during **QS**, but these dreams are usually fragmentary - one image or scene.

After 40 to 80 minutes of sleep, you enter the second sleep state, **Active Sleep (AS)**. During **AS** your brain waves speed up, the muscle tension at your chin decreases, you have body twitches, your breathing becomes shallow, your heart rate speeds up, your blood pressure varies, men may have penile erection, your thoughts become dream-like and dramatic, and you commence **Rapid Eye Movements (REM's)** - that is, your eyes begin to dart around under your closed eyelids at a rapid pace 3 to 5 times a night in 20 minute segments. Our dreams during **AS** are detailed action sequences. In general, **AS** segments increase in duration as the night progresses.

Contrary to popular opinion, most of our dreams are not bizarre or unusual; but are very commonplace experiences. They include another person; but seldom an animal. Most are active but not strenuous, such as talking or walking. The length of a dream is about the same as the time it would take to imagine it awake - for seconds or minutes.

There is no reliable explanation for the meaning of dreams; but they are believed to represent a broad range of concerns rather than one, such as sexuality.

We do not know why we dream, or what dreams mean; but we do know that people deprived of **AS** and the accompanying dreams suffer no behavioral problems.

Two needs served by **AS** dreaming though are the consolidation of memories, and the assimilation of traumatic experiences. If there is no **AS** dreaming, there is no long term memory. That is why cramming before an exam without sleeping does not work.

Much research has been done on the subject of learning during sleep, and the research clearly shows that it is not possible to learn complicated material during sleep.

Although total time spent asleep is the same in various age groups, some changes do occur in sleep patterns as we age:

1. Older persons take longer to fall asleep than do the young.
2. Older persons awaken more frequently during the night and spend a longer time awake on each occasion. The older person thus spends longer total time in bed.
3. The transition between sleep and wakefulness is abrupt in older people in contrast with the period of "coming to the surface" that young people go through. Older people are thus considered "light sleepers".
4. Older people go into **AS** less and less, and awaken more frequently and for longer periods of time.
5. There is a sharp reduction in dream recall with aging.
6. Penile erections during **AS** are reduced by as much as 50% in the much older man.

The most beneficial sleep habit is to sleep at the same time every day, in the same place, wearing the same clothing if any, and in the same company. The more regular the schedule and familiar the surroundings, the more relaxed will be the sleep; and therefore the more restful.

It is also easiest to fall asleep at the same time each day, and in familiar surroundings. If one does have difficulty falling asleep, it helps to think of relaxing each part of the body, beginning with the toes and moving up the body until finally the mind is cleared and made to try to think of nothing at all.

If sleep still does not come, it may help to get up and do something for a short time (nothing strenuous or stimulating); perhaps have a glass of warm milk (it contains the amino acid Tryptophane, which promotes sleep) or other non-caffeine beverage, then try again. A glass of wine with dinner sometimes relaxes one enough to prepare them for sleep later, as does a sexual release. Silence and darkness are both helpful in falling asleep.

All responsible research reported to date regarding sleep aids (drugs) points ever more dramatically in the same direction: sleeping pills and other forms of drugs used to induce sleep deteriorate the system dramatically. The conclusion is clear: don't use them unless prescribed by your doctor; and then we recommend getting a second opinion. Sleep-inducing drugs are prescribed much too often by doctors, according to recent studies. Habitual users of sleeping pills could add at least five more healthy years to their lives by discontinuing the use of such pills and drugs.

People who now have irregular sleeping habits could add at least another five healthy years to their lives by getting at least seven hours of sleep every night, at about the same time each night. Those who already get a full night's sleep every night could add at least five more healthy years of life by making it a practice of napping for at least half an hour each noon.

Be aware that, no matter what you may have heard or read, we still do not know the exact nature of sleep, or exactly what goes on during this physical and mental process. That is the reason that dreams still cannot be interpreted with any certainty of accuracy. There are people who speak convincingly about what a particular dream might mean, but their speculations are not likely to be any more accurate than yours.

Carl Bourhenne, MA
Gerontologist

Carl Bourhenne's

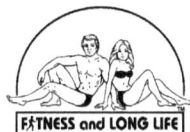

FITNESS and LONG LIFE

How To Live
The Longest Life Possible

Psychological
Do What You <u>Like</u> To Do, Expectations

Have a positive attitude toward life. <u>**Expect**</u> **to live a
long time.** <u>**Find out what you like to do, and do it!**</u>

The first indication that a positive attitude toward life is a
big asset toward a healthy long life came   from   a
forty year long study initiated in 1937, at   Harvard
University. The study showed that
the participants who were most
pessimistic at age 25 had many more
serious illnesses in their sixties.

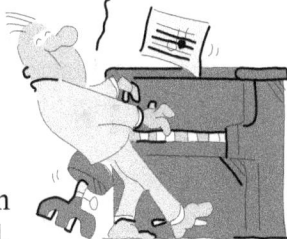

The newly emerging field in
medicine of the discipline called,
"psychoneuroimmunology" continues to impress researchers.
Ever since cancer treatments began to successfully use
"visioning" to encourage patients to mentally fight their
cancer, the medical community's interest in a positive
attitude for health has grown. The reason that having a
positive attitude toward life promotes a healthy long life is
that the immune system, our protector of life, is physically

linked to the nervous system. In fact, our sympathetic nervous system (SNS) continually exercises control over the immune system.

When we are in an up, or positive frame of mind the immune system is stimulated by the SNS. But when we are down because of stress or depression the immune system is suppressed by the SNS. For example, negative personal situations such as loneliness have been shown to suppress cancer-fighting NK white blood cells.

And the body of data has been growing, so that this relatively new field of psychoneuroimmunology is being adopted into the medical schools.

Having a positive attitude toward life affects more than just the immune system, though. When we think positive thoughts we generate a shower of supportive hormones, endorphins, and other chemicals that stimulate our systems into activity, and thus health.

Having too many or prolonged negative thoughts and attitudes, however, generates showers of inhibitive hormones and chemicals into the system, slowing it down and impairing our functioning and our health. So it truly pays to have a positive attitude toward life.

Just as positive thinking stimulates our system, our expectations prepare our systems for what is to come. If we **expect** to live a long life, the expectation itself stimulates our system to generate health promoting hormones and other chemicals, just as our expectation of seeing a loved one stimulates all of the chemicals that cause our pulse to race and our attitude to soar.

If we expect to live a long life, we will tend more to internally prepare for and provide for a long, healthy life.

The directive, **"<u>Find out what you like to do and do it</u>"** goes hand in hand with the reasons stated above for having a positive attitude toward life. Having to continually force ourselves to do what we don't particularly enjoy or despise can only slow our systems, including our immune system, and lead to poor health and a shorter lifespan.

Doing something that we find enjoyable though, stimulates our entire system, enlivening and invigorates us, promoting a healthy long life.

There is also evidence that ambivalence about goals and directions is unhealthy. One who is ambivalent about what they want to do tends to analyze more and act less, and the results of such ambivalence and inactivity can be chest pains, dizziness, nausea, headaches, and depression.

For some of us, finding out what we like to do and doing it requires great effort. Just finding out what we like to do requires much thought and self-assessment, and is perhaps the most difficult task of all. Often a friend or counselor can help, and the process of discovery could take weeks, months, or even longer.

But once this discovery is made, life takes on new meaning, and everything seems possible.

Carl Bourhenne, MA
Gerontologist

126

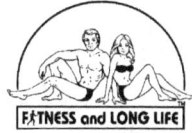

How To Live
The Longest Life Possible

Medical Care
And
Transplants, Bionics, Biological Youth Treatments

Have regular health checkups. See a doctor when you detect a problem. Follow a doctor's advice when taking medications.

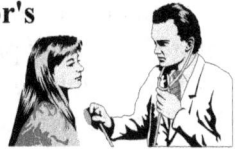

B y now it is common knowledge that the best defense against major health disaster is early detection and early treatment. And the regular health checkup, if extensive and of good quality, is the most consistent means to early detection. The American Cancer Society in particular stresses the vital importance of regular health checkups for early detection and early treatment.

But how frequent, and how extensive should our health checkups be? The general guideline is that the older we get, the more frequent and the more extensive our health checkups should be.

From a cost-for-return point of view, annual physicals **before the age of about 30** might not be necessary. Immediate action in response to suspicious symptoms might be adequate until that time.

Between the ages of 30 to 40, complaint-free individuals and those not taking any medication should have a physical examination every five years.

Between the ages of about 40 to 50, a physical examination is recommended every three years.

Between the ages of 50 to 60, a physical examination is recommended every two years.

After 60, an annual physical is recommended.

Everyone might have their teeth cleaned and cared for every three to six months. Of course, at any age, unusual symptoms should be investigated immediately.

Also, there are certain circumstances under which physical examinations should be performed:
-Women should always have a physical examination before becoming pregnant.
-Anyone taking medications, including women on the Pill, should have annual physical
   examinations.

In addition, there are specific items that should be checked regularly:
   ♥-- Everyone should have a blood pressure check at least
       every two years.
   ♥-- A **TB Test** should be **every three to five years**; and
       if you have been exposed to TB, it should be taken
       every year.
   ♥-- A Pap test **(Pap smear)** **every 6 to 12 months** to
       screen for cervical cancer -- completely curable if
       caught early.
   ♥-- A **glaucoma test** (for pressure inside the eyeball,
       which leads to blindness) should be administered

every two years after 35.

♥-- People between the **ages of 30 to 50**, should be
screened for bowel cancer every two years; and from
the **age of 50 on**, every year.

See A Doctor When You Detect A Problem!

The determination of whether or not to see a doctor is not
always an easy one to make. There are such a variety of
circumstances and conditions which might call for such
action that they could not possibly all be addressed here, but
**there are certain conditions which should be attended to
immediately:**

Heart attacks: The number of people who die each year
could be greatly reduced by seeking medical care
immediately, rather than delaying for hours.

Cancer: Early detection and treatment could reduce the
number of deaths each year.

Massive bleeding that cannot be stopped.

Major burns

Possible broken bones

Poisoning, or suspected poisoning.

Severe pain

Cold sweats, especially if accompanied by light-headedness,
or chest or abdominal pain.

Severe shortness of breath (if not due to exertion).

Unconsciousness, stupor, or disorientation as to time,
place, or name.

Running fever for more than a week

A lump in the breast.

Unexplained weight loss

Coughing up blood

Blood in the stool or urine.

Any physical problem which persists for an unusual period
of time.

If you are told by a doctor that you need surgery, always get a second opinion.

Follow A Doctor's Advice When Taking Medications

The first precept in dealing with your doctor regarding medications is to advise your doctor of any medications you are already taking, and of any allergies that you might have.

Once your doctor has prescribed medication for you to take, use the following guidelines to assure that you have all of the information that you need to follow your doctor's advice in taking them:

Know what the drug is, both brand name and generic name.
Know what the drug is supposed to do.
Know precisely how you are to take the drug (swallowed, inhaled, etc.; with water, etc.).
Know when to take the drug (how often, with meals, etc.).
Are lifestyle changes required (no alcohol, don't drive etc.).
How long to take the drug (take all of them?, until the symptoms disappear?, etc.).
What to do if you miss a dose.
What side effects to expect.
What the drug will cost, and if you can buy a generic.

Remember, if your doctor prescribes a drug, fill it and take it. **Never** take a drug prescribed for someone else, and **always** throw out old medications.

Before proceeding further, I will point out the need for each one of us to keep an eye on our own bodies in order to treat problems at the earliest possible moment. This can very often be the difference between life and death:

Self - Examinations

Self - Examinations might be a regular process for each of us - men and women. I will not delve here into each of

130

the many self - exam techniques for men and women.

Once you have concluded that you do need professional medical help, the first step is to select the individual with whom you will entrust the care of your body. The most important factor here is to make sure that you go to a medical doctor first, then accept referrals to other specialists.

To provide you with some basic guidelines in evaluating a doctor for yourself, I offer the following check list:

1) Is the staff in the doctor's office warm and interested, or busy and hurried? You should be made welcome and comfortable.

2) Does the staff answer all your questions? You should not be left to wonder about anything.

3) When you call, are you put through to the doctor when you ask to speak with him?

4) Is the waiting room comfortable and cheerful, or crowded, not well decorated, or uncomfortable? Are you kept informed of delays?

5) Does the doctor take a complete medical history on your first visit? Does he show a general interest in your well-being, as well as in your present problem?

6) Does he use jargon, or words that you, as a layperson understand? Is he obese? Does he smoke? Is he a good listener?

7) Are the purposes of all tests explained to you? Is the equipment modern, or shopworn?

8) While talking with the doctor, does he put you at ease, and encourage questions? Does he preach, talk down, give orders, or speak quickly? Does he summarize his findings, explain his conclusions, and encourage you to call in a few days whenever you feel the need?

Even when you, after self-examination, detect no medical problems, and have no immediate, noticeable need of medical care, you should make your regular check-ups one of the most important commitments to yourself.

Even a check-up every six months is not a waste of time, and even every three months if there is any history or pre-disposition to cancer in your family.

Are you thinking of the cost? How much would you be willing to pay for an additional month, or year of life; or of being youthful, healthy, and attractive instead of incapacitated and/or hospitalized? How much would you pay for five years, or ten years? Of what use will the money be if you are not here?

Transplants

Transplants, or "spare parts surgery" as it is becoming known, is giving many additional years of life to many people who are healthy except for, perhaps one body part. Often these people are young, attractive, and active; or could be active and normal if only that one body part could be successfully replaced (assuming it cannot be repaired).

Many people are presently receiving replacement body parts from donors but the pervading problems continue to be availability of organs, and rejection of these transplanted parts by the immune system of the recipient. The immune system must reject invaders, or germs and disease would enter and run rampant throughout the body.

The job of the immune system is to destroy and reject all invaders. The transplanted body part is recognized as an invader, so it attacks the transplanted body part. Procedures have been developed to suppress the recipient's immune system, but if it is suppressed too much, then germs and disease will run rampant, and eventually kill the recipient of the transplant. Research continues, of course, to solve this serious problem; but a problem it remains.

The most prominent successes in transplants are seen in cases where the donor's blood type and biological make-up are most similar to that of the recipient, so that the transplanted part is more acceptable to the recipient's immune system. If the donor was biologically identical to the recipient, there would be no rejection and the transplant would be successful, barring other types of complications.

The better successes have been with transplants between relatives, the closer the better, because of the biological similarities. In fact, the best successes have been with transplants between identical twins. Since they are biologically identical, there is no rejection factor.

The art and science of "spare parts surgery" has come a long way since the first real kidney transplant in 1949 by David Hume, from Harvard Medical School. Since then over 57,000 kidney transplants have been performed, and many people are alive today as a result of them. Over 190 lung transplants have been performed, over 590 heart transplants, over 475 liver transplants, about 350 pancreas transplants, well over 350 bone transplants since the discovery that the immune system will accept bone transplants if the bone is frozen, then thawed; over 10,500 cornea transplants, with a very good success rate.

The serious problem of rejection of transplanted parts, however, still prevents the transplant operation from being the complete solution for those who could continue normal life with the replacement of some one worn or damaged body part.

The ideal donor is someone who is biologically identical to the recipient (such as an identical twin), and that in this way there is no rejection factor. Unfortunately, we do not all have an identical twin and so perhaps the future most promising, but morally debated method of obtaining spare body parts for yourself is the actual growing of your own spare body parts for yourself, from your own cells.

This process is called "limited cloning" of yourself. By this method, you might live much longer than is presently possible because you would have a full complement of spare body parts for yourself, with no rejection factor.

In "limited cloning" you are cloned, but only your vital body parts are allowed to develop. As we mentioned above, this process is a hotly debated moral issue. As yet, contrary to some sensational publications, no human has ever been cloned; only organisms such as frogs have been successfully cloned. The process is so well founded in scientific research though, that modern scientists say that it is only a matter of time before human cloning is technologically possible. The difficulty has been in the delicacy of the human egg in withstanding the injection of a new nucleus.

Bionics

The most important advantage of bionic implants at this time, is that bionic organs and limbs, when implanted, are not usually rejected by the body's immune system. The immune system recognizes only proteins, and bionics are not made of proteins, but of synthetic materials.

The word "Bionics" was coined from the Greek words "BIOS" (life), and "ICS" (having the nature of), in September of 1960 by a meeting of scientists.

A Bionic organ or limb is one which is artificial, but is implanted or biologically attached to the recipient's body, and has electronic controlling devices.

Some of the bionic body parts which have been successfully developed and used to date are:
Bionic Limbs (arms and legs)   Heart Valves

Blood	Seeing Devices
Kidneys	Hearing Devices
Pancreas	Bones
Heart	Joints
Liver	Ligaments
Lungs	Muscles
Tendons	

And, even bionic Erection Assistance Devices, in which artificial valves in the male genitalia are implanted to replace non-functioning valves. The erections are real, the valves are simply replacements of natural valves which ceased to function.

These bionic parts are made of synthetic materials and utilize electronics, electric motors, and miniature battery systems. In some cases the motor switches are connected directly to nerves, and use the natural electric output of the nerve itself to start and control the motorized bionic part. These are called "myoelectric limbs", which are actually "thought" into action by the brain.

Bionics is considered by scientists to be a fascinating field with a rapidly growing future. The Society of Biomaterials was formed in 1972, and other supportive activities are being formulated to advance the art and science of bionics for better living, longer.

Biological Youth Treatments

The most popular current "youth treatments" being offered in various health resorts for the rich around the world, and details regarding their application and effectiveness are described in detail in the following pages.

The five most popular biological youth treatments are:
  1) Plasmapheresis

2) Estrogen Therapy
3) Cell Therapy
4) The "Youth Pill"
5) Regeneresen Therapy

1) Plasmapheresis

B ased on the concept that the blood is the supplier of life and the cleanser of the body, Dr. Norman Orentreich, one of America's most renowned plastic surgeons and dermatologists, began experiments on this process in 1964 using laboratory animals. In 1966 he began experiments on a human volunteer, and observers say that the sixty year old man has the appearance of a much younger man. Once per week the man arrived at Dr. Orentreich's clinic in New York. Two pints of his blood were withdrawn from his arm and processed through a machine by centrifugal spinning, at below freezing temperature. The red blood cells were separated from the plasma. The red cells were then returned to the man's body, minus the plasma. The process took about 90 minutes. The belief is that, along with the plasma, the "aging acceleration factors" (the toxic effects of metabolism) are thus removed from the blood.

There is not sufficient evidence at this time to support a conclusion as to whether or not plasmapheresis is truly a preserver of youth. You may wish to experiment yourself, and if you are so disposed, the opportunity may be readily accessible to you. Your local blood bank might accept donations of platelets only, for leukemia victims. This is done by withdrawing 2 pints of your blood, then returning the red blood cells to your body. They might, however, try to talk you into simply donating your whole blood instead of just the platelets, since the plasmapheresis process is more troublesome. This, of course, would not accomplish your objective.

2) Estrogen Therapy

This treatment is performed by a physician prescribing supplements of the female hormone, estrogen.

It is used primarily to help ease some women through menopause and after, and is grossly over-used - mainly because so many women today have an enormously overrated view of its potential merits. Less than 50% of women in menopause can benefit from estrogen therapy. The rest will encounter no benefit, and may well experience extremely unpleasant and unhealthy side effects. We must not overlook the fact, though, that to some women estrogen therapy does provide great relief from severe menopausal and post-menopausal distress.

The reason for the over-use and abuse of estrogen therapy is a result of the determination of some women to either talk their reluctant doctor into prescribing it, or go from doctor to doctor until they find one who will prescribe it.

The average age of the onset of menses is now about twelve years, and the average age of beginning the twelve to thirty-six month stage of menopause is just over fifty years; and this may be delayed by a daily injection of 100 IU. of vitamin E three times per day.

The best means of controlling tension, anxiety, and emotional balance during menopause is an excellent diet, and most especially, regular exercise programs.

Only after proper lifestyle habits have been applied to one's daily life, should a patient or her doctor even consider estrogen therapy, and then the doctor's decision (perhaps after a second opinion) should be accepted. And this decision should not be finalized as a result of testing for estrogen levels, since there are no dependable tests known at this time which will provide an accurate reading of estrogen levels. The readings of estrogen levels are often strongly affected by the offsetting action of progesterone in the system.

Research has shown that prolonged periods of estrogen therapy can be damaging to the health. If the patient has been taking birth control pills, she has already had exposure to estrogen therapy. The best and the healthiest way to raise the estrogen levels, and thus receive increased benefits to health and attractiveness, is through an exercise regimen which should be accompanied by a nutrition and diet program.

3) Cell Therapy

The process of injecting into people, the cells - either fresh or quick-frozen (fresh are preferred), - of shredded sheep organs into the buttocks, has been offered by rejuvenation centers around the world since the 1940's. My research turned up many reports of favorable results, but without controlled tests or post-treatment results-measuring exams. So, there are no confirmed reports of favorable results, and no scientific reason to accept cell therapy as a valid rejuvenating method in and of itself.

Cell therapy treatment is followed by a period of rest, then good nutrition and exercise.

The follow-up procedures all by themselves are very rejuvenating, but there is no conclusive evidence that cell therapy really works, in spite of the numerous and vociferous supporters who espouse its wondrous effects against old age. Perhaps that is the reason the process is not approved by the American Medical Association, and is not legal in the United States.

4) The Youth Pill
(Gerovital)

Procaine, a relative of the drug Novocain, is the chemical base for the "youth pill", a product of Dr. Ana Aslan of Romania.   Dr. Aslan is director of the Bucharest Geriatric Institute, and developer of the "youth pill", also known as H-3, GH-3, or KH-3 when a blood derivative called "hematorporphyrin" is added in an attempt to make the oral version as effective as the injection is said to be.

Another common name for this "youth pill", is "Gerovital". The claimed benefits are very many indeed, and the number of people around the world who claim to have received benefits from the "youth pill" are very, very numerous.   This is not surprising, since its base is a derivative of a major drug. No impressive results have ever been seen in any legitimate geriatric study, and special U.S. Government authorization is required to import the KH-3 capsules.

Most of the known "youth doctors" around the world deny any significant effectiveness of the "youth pill".   They suggest that the most important factor for the belief by people in the effectiveness of this type of product is the belief itself. A belief, itself, in a youth product causes those using it to take much better care of themselves, and the better care itself is an effective youth treatment.

5) Regeneresen Therapy

This "youth treatment", also known as "RNA Therapy", is based on the concept that, as we grow older the RNA (ribonucleic acid) in our cells gradually loses its ability to accurately direct the production of the various kinds of protein necessary to sustain our life. This treatment was developed by Dr. Benjamin S. Frank, in New York. Dr. Frank proposed three methods for RNA therapy:

1. **Dietary**
2. **Supplemental**
3. **Organ-specific**

1. **The Dietary Method** simply consists of increasing the intake of foods that Dr. Frank has concluded are rich in nucleic acids: Liver, kidneys, anchovies, sweetbreads, sardines, and meat and fish extracts.
2. **The Supplemental Method** consists of eating RNA supplements, refined from yeast.
3. **The Organ-specific Method** consists of injecting into ourselves the RNA from whichever animal organ is weak in ourselves.

For example, if our liver is weak we inject into ourselves the RNA taken from the liver of an animal, and thus also the heart, kidney, etc.

There is no convincing substantiation for these treatments. In fact, any form of RNA or DNA which is ingested orally is entirely destroyed by the digestive system, and none of it is utilized as planned.

Carl Bourhenne, MA
Gerontologist

Carl Bourhenne's

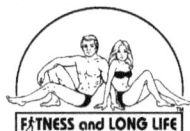

How To Live
The Longest Life Possible

Safety Factors
Driving

Use Seatbelts. Practice good safety habits at home to prevent accidents such as fires and falls. Many people suddenly lose their lives, and many more lose aspects of their health due to accidents. It is so unfortunate for someone to suddenly lose the remaining ten, thirty, fifty or more years of their life; or lose their ability to move around on their own, all because of a quick, unexpected accident.

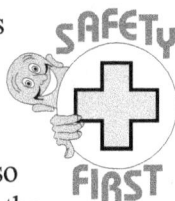

The following tips are designed to make sure that such a thing does not happen to you:

<u>Use Seatbelts:</u> In 1996 there were 57,038 deaths due to motor vehicle accidents. This represents people from the following age groups:

AGE	DEATHS
Under 14	6,466
15-24	20,650
25 +	16,112

Automobile accidents are the fourth leading cause of death in the United States, after heart disease, cancer, and stroke. In fact, **more people died as a result of motor vehicle accidents in 1978 (50,000) than Americans who died in World War I, the Korean War, or all ten years of the Vietnam conflict, <u>combined</u>!**

Motor vehicle accidents kill, cripple, and change the lives of more people than any other kind of accident. **The motor vehicle is the leading cause of accidental deaths of people under 75 years of age, and the leading cause of all deaths of people between the ages of 15 and 24.**

75% of automobile deaths are males, and most do not involve other vehicles (accidents involving overturning, running off the road, and running into stationary objects).

Almost half of teenage deaths involve excessive speed (44%). Accidents of those 75 years old and over tend to involve right-of-way violations, such as disregard of traffic control, failure to yield, and pedestrian accidents. **A disproportionate number of traffic fatalities occur at night.**

<u>One-half of all motor vehicle accidents involve alcohol.</u> 62% of all deaths and injuries involving alcohol occur between 6 P.M. and 3 A.M. <u>There has been a sharp increase in traffic accidents since the lowering of the drinking age</u>. Avoid dangerous situations in traffic. Follow all traffic laws (there are good reasons for each one), drive defensively, and watch out for pedestrians.

<u>Some practical rules for driving safety are:</u>
1. Keep your driving speed within the posted limits.
2. Obey all traffic laws; carefully avoid minor traffic violations.
3. Don't sneak through yellow lights.

4. Signal well in advance of turning.
1. Maintain proper distance from the vehicle in front.
2. Follow all speed control regulations.

Neglecting just <u>one</u> of these precautions <u>once,</u> can cost a life or a limb.

Home Safety Tips

Prevent Fires: Practice good safety habits at home to prevent accidents such as fires and falls. Accidents touch the lives of more people than any other type of trauma.   And surprisingly, the United States leads the world in deaths caused by fires. In fact, 8,000 people are killed in home fires each year, and 300,000 people are injured. One house in 16 will have a fire this year.

This data is important only to bring each of us to the awareness that fires in the home are an imminent danger to each of us - not just to "the other guy".

Here are some additional statistics, just to let you know what to look out for:

Fires in the bedroom and the living room are the most dangerous, although only about one fourth of all fires start there. They account for 7 out of 10 home fire deaths.

Almost two thirds of all home fires start in the kitchen, but result in only 1 in 6 deaths.

75% of fatal home fires start between 9:00 P.M. and 7:00 A.M.

75% of home fire deaths are due to fumes and hypoxia (lack of oxygen), not burning.

You might want to note these preventive measures to help prevent a fire in your home:
1.   Buy and install smoke detectors.

2. Design and practice a fire drill procedure for your family.
3. Keep flammable items clear of fire hazards and electrical dangers.
4. Don't place individual room heaters too close to draperies or furniture, where they might start a fire.
5. Inspect fuel-burning furnaces regularly. Clogged flues may allow dangerous gasses to accumulate inside the house.
6. Have fireplace chimneys inspected and cleaned annually to prevent buildup of creosote, a material that may catch fire.
7. If you smoke, **don't smoke in bed**.

In the unfortunate event that you have a fire, follow these important guidelines to safety:
1) Follow your pre-planned fire drill procedure.
2) Roll out of bed (don't jump up), to stay below the smoke and toxic gasses.
3) Aim to get out of the house immediately. Don't stop to pick up valuables. Don't reach for the phone. Don't get dressed. Just get out. You can quickly be overcome by smoke.
4) Crawl toward your primary fire exit (usually the door) on your hands and knees, not on your belly. Some toxic gasses are heavy, and settle near the floor.
5) When you get to the door, don't open it immediately. Feel the doorknob. If it's hot, don't open it; find another way out. If it's not hot, open it; if you're met with smoke, close it immediately and find another way out.
6) Close every door behind you (but don't lock any), to suppress drafts from feeding the fire.
7) If your clothes catch on fire, don't run. Lie down and roll the fire out.
8) Never go back into a burning building.

9) Replace damaged or worn electrical cords.
10) Never run electrical cords across rooms, or under rugs or other objects.
11) When using electrical appliances, follow all directions.
12) Don't overload house circuits.

Home Safety

1. Be sure, when using electrical appliances, that your hands are dry and that you are standing on a dry floor.
2. Use plastic instead of glass containers in the bathroom.
3. Put non-skid pads in the tub and shower.
4. Never leave an infant unattended in the bath, even for a moment.
5. Make sure you have quick access to your main controls for gas, water, and electricity.
6. Store heavy items low to the floor.
7. Wrap razor blades and broken glass well before discarding.
8. Use a stepladder rather than furniture to climb to high places.
9. Clean the oven of excess grease, and don't leave greasy pans or aluminum inside.
10. You may have an unwanted fire if you forget they are there and light the oven.
11. Lock up sharp objects such as scissors and tools, especially electrical tools, from children.
12. Inspect your stove and other gas appliances regularly for leaks.
13. Lock up your power lawn mower, and don't try to refuel a hot engine.
14. Make sure all windows lock, for security at night.
15. Maintain a complete first aid kit.
17. Keep the right kinds of fire extinguishers in the right places. Your fire department can help.
17. Make sure that any hooks, etc. are above eye level.
18. Make certain that sliding glass doors are visible, and

have shatterproof glass.

19. Put emergency phone numbers readily visible on the phone: Fire Dept., Police, Ambulance, and your local Poison Control Center (see the white pages).
20. Beware of wearing loose clothing near gas burners.
21. Always remove your car keys from the car.
22. Stairway light switches should be both at the top and at the bottom of the stairway.
23. Lift objects with your legs, not your back, and always get help when moving heavy objects.

Special Safety Tips For Seniors

Many "broken hips" in the elderly are not really broken hips, but "femoral neck fractures". That is, the neck of the femur bone, in the area of the hip becomes weak due to osteoporosis and breaks. Too often the resulting immobilization results in death not long after the accident. For this reason it is imperative that precautions be taken to lessen the likelihood of such an accident.

The following suggestions may help:

♥ Make certain that all carpet edges are tacked down to avoid tripping.
♥ Do not leave toys or other items in walkways.
♥ Have hand rails installed in the bathroom to aid balance.
♥ Check all steps and stairways for adequate light, handrails, and resting places.
♥ Make certain that all walking pathways are firm, and not slippery.
♥ Have all medications in childproof containers, with large lettering.

Carl Bourhenne, MA
Gerontologist

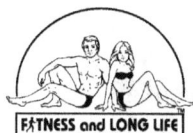

How To Live
The Longest Life Possible

Financial Security

Plan ahead for Housing, Medical, and Financial Security

SAVE MONEY!

So often I am asked what the one, single, most important factor is in living a long, healthy life. The question is inevitably followed by a suggested answer, usually either "Exercise" or "Nutrition". Many longevity researchers will say that the single most important factor for a healthy long life, youthful and attractive is...surprise!...Having a lot of money!

The reason that this is the answer often given is that without enough money to provide the healthy necessities of life, the free time to exercise and do all of the things that promote optimum health and attractiveness, and the financial resources to live a relatively stress free lifestyle, optimum health is difficult to attain.

While some poorer people like to believe that people with money are unhappy, nothing could be further from the truth.

Everyone has problems of one kind or another, and a certain percentage of every population are essentially unhappy. But for most people, the more money they have the more likely they are to be and to perceive themselves as happy, just as you and I are happier now than we would be if we had less money.

Furthermore, the more money that we have, the more able we are to live a stress free lifestyle, eat right, and have time to exercise and do all of the other fulfilling activities that make us healthy, youthful, and attractive for a longer life.

The heading of this section urges us to plan ahead for housing and financial security. It is critically important that we arrange our finances in such a manner that we will have all of the means to provide ourselves with housing, good food, medical care, and the opportunities for exercise, social activities, and all of the other factors that promote a healthy long life. We certainly must make provisions for an adequate living, and set aside or invest for that time when we will not work for our income.

The purpose of this section is not to design a financial program for you. There is not enough space here, and that can only be done by a Certified Financial Planner who can talk to you about where you will want to live, what your interests and hobbies are and will be, and what you anticipate your future interests will be.

Be aware of the importance of housing, medical, and financial needs for a healthy long life, and to cheer you on in your pursuit of your financial and material goals.

The more money you can obtain the better you can provide for ways to live a stress free life, full of the wide variety of factors that are generally necessary for the longest life, healthy, youthful, and attractive.

The research clearly shows that no single group of persons lives as long as those with a lot of money, for the reasons stated above. It is for these reasons that I encourage you to combine the fact that the self-employed are among the longest living (self-employment is one of the two lowest stress occupations because one has no supervisors), with the fact that the self-employed also generally have the best opportunity to make a lot of money.

Perhaps self-employment is not for you, and if it is not, then it is not best for your healthy long life.

But if self-employment is for you, then you have a dual opportunity to realize the most of your 120 possible years of life.

The most important message that this section holds for you though is, indeed, to plan ahead for housing, medical, and financial security. And the best way to do this is to **hire a Certified Financial Planner who does not sell stocks or insurance, or any other items or services**.

Pay the financial planner for planning and strategy only, and do not use his or her services in any other capacity, and do not use the services of any persons that he or she recommends. Go elsewhere for such recommendations to avoid serious conflicts of interests that could cost you very dearly, indeed.

If the Certified (make sure he or she is Certified) Financial Planner pushes you to buy or do anything else from or through him or her, then leave and find someone else. Few stock brokers are Certified Financial Planners, and even if yours is, does it seem wise to let them talk you into doing your financial planning while they are trying to sell you investment instruments such as stocks and bonds? Perhaps not.

And now, perhaps as important as anything else that this section can say is: **Make certain that you always have good Medical Insurance!**

It can unexpectedly make the difference between life and death and, as importantly, the regular check-ups alone could save your life.

Carl Bourhenne, MA
Gerontologist

Carl Bourhenne's

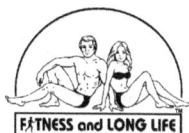

FITNESS and LONG LIFE

How To Live
The Longest Life Possible

Environmental Concerns

Avoid overexposure to the sun and cold. The body's ability to regulate and monitor its own temperature seems to decline with age, making the elderly more vulnerable to heat and cold stress.

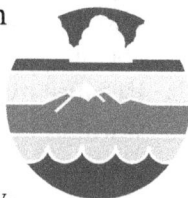

Hypothermia is a condition of below-normal body temperature - typically 95øF (35øC) or under, and can be fatal. Accidental hypothermia may occur in anyone who is exposed to severe cold without enough protection. However, some older people can develop accidental hypothermia after exposure to relatively mild cold. For unknown reasons, some older people do not feel cold and do not shiver. Thus, they cannot produce body heat by shivering when they need it. It is interesting to note that many people who have "felt cold" for years may actually have a lower risk of accidental hypothermia.

The only sure way to detect hypothermia is to use a special low-reading thermometer, available in most hospitals; but a regular thermometer will do if you shake it down well. If the temperature is below 95øF (35øC) or does not register, call for emergency medical help.

Other signs to look for include: An unusual change in appearance or behavior during cold weather; slow, and sometimes irregular heartbeat; slurred speech; shallow, very slow breathing; sluggishness and confusion. Treatment consists of re-warming the person under a doctor's supervision, preferably in a hospital.

Protective Measures Against Hypothermia:
In cold weather: There is no strong scientific basis for recommending specific room temperatures. However, setting the heat at 65øF (18.3øC) in living and sleeping areas should be adequate in most cases, although sick people may need more heat.

Measures To Prevent Accidental Hypothermia Include:
1) Dress warmly, even when indoors. Eat enough food, and stay as active as possible.
2) Because hypothermia may start even during sleep, keep warm in bed by wearing enough clothing and using blankets.
3) If you take medicine to treat anxiety, depression, nervousness, or nausea, ask your doctor whether the medication might affect the control of body temperature.
4) If you stay alone, especially in later years, ask friends or neighbors to look in on you once or twice a day, particularly during a cold spell. See if your community has a telephone check-in or personal visit service for the elderly or home-bound.

Heat Effects And H eat-Related Illnesses: The major heat-related illnesses are Heat Stroke, and Heat Exhaustion.

Heat Stroke is a medical emergency requiring immediate attention and treatment by a doctor. Among the symptoms

152

are faintness, dizziness, headache, nausea, loss of consciousness, body temperature of 104øF (40øC) or higher, measured rectally, rapid pulse, and flushed skin.

Heat Exhaustion takes longer to develop than other heat-related illnesses. It results from a loss of body water and salt. The symptoms include weakness, heavy sweating, nausea, and giddiness. Heat Exhaustion is treated by resting in bed away from the heat, and drinking cool liquids.

Protective measures for hot weather:
The ideal place to be during hot spells is indoors, in an air-conditioned room. If your home is not air-conditioned, you might go to a cool public place like a library, movie theater, or store during the hottest hours.

Other good ways to cool off include taking cool baths or showers, placing ice-bags or wet towels on the body, and using electric fans.

It also wise to do the following:
-Stay out of direct sunlight and avoid strenuous activity during heat spells. (Cells from sun-exposed skin divide fewer times in culture than unexposed cells, indicating a possible speeding up of the aging process by the sun's rays.
-Wear light-weight, light-colored, loose-fitting clothing that permits sweat to evaporate.
-Drink plenty of liquids such as water, fruit and vegetable juice, and iced tea to replace the fluids lost by sweating. Try not to drink alcoholic beverages or fluids that have too much salt, since salt can complicate existing medical problems, such as high blood pressure. Use salt tablets only with your doctor's approval.

Above all, take the heat seriously and don't ignore danger signs like nausea, dizziness, and fatigue.

The main Environmental Factors that affect our healthy Long Life are:
1. Our Geographic Location
2. The Temperature in our Home
3. Our Safety Habits

   1. <u>**Your Geographic Location**</u>: Although all of the reasons are not clearly understood, there is no doubt that the length of our life varies considerably from one region to another. Some of the reasons are the purity and content of the air, the water, the climate, the mineral content of the soil, the altitude, and, **most significantly of all - our way of life.** <u>Some notable facts of interest in this regard are</u>: Those who live in a State in the Rocky Mountain Time Zone, or in New Mexico, Alaska, or Hawaii tend to live three to six years longer than people in other parts of the United States.

   Those who live in small towns tend to live four to eight years longer than people who live in a city of a million or more people.

   If you live in a city of a million or more people, you can take these steps to reduce your own exposure to stress and pollution:

   <u>**First**</u>, try to be relaxed and easy-going. Try to have fun in everything you do including work, and laugh a lot of conflicts off - then, <u>never hold a grudge (forgive easily)</u>.

   <u>**Second**</u>, protect yourself as much as possible from the chemicals and pollutants of a large city.
   <u>**Third, and most important,**</u> get a lot of exercise and strenuous activity. Strenuous exercise plays a very large part in keeping the immune system strong to fight viruses, which are more abundant in larger populated areas.

The ideal geographic situation, and the conditions in which people live the healthiest and longest lives seem to be in **hilly country, with no mechanical means of transportation,** and only natural foods, such as in the three areas where there is an unusually large number of centenarians:

1) The Abkhasians in the Caucasus Mountains of Soviet Georgia.

2) The Vilcabambans in the Ecuadorian Andes.

3) The Hunzas in the Karakorum Mountains of Kashmir in West Pakistan's Himalayas.

2 . Temperature Control: Research has repeatedly shown that a lower temperature in the home produces a significantly longer life span. Experiments with some organisms have shown that living in lower temperatures doubles the life spans of those organisms (rotifers, etc.). 68ø is a healthier temperature to maintain in the home than is 72ø, especially early in life; but does remain significant throughout life. Lower temperatures inhibit the proliferation of bacteria, and reduce wear and tear on the human organism, slowing down the aging process.

3 . Safety Habits
Obviously, we must move about in our lives with an awareness of intelligent safety precautions against injury from accidents if we want to live long, healthy lives. The most significant factor in this regard is safety on the streets while driving motor vehicles.
Driving accidents are the cause of so many disabilities, injuries, and deaths each year, that driving safety is a definite factor in long life.
Some Practical Rules For Driving Safety Are:
1) Keep your driving speed within the posted limits.

2) Obey all traffic laws; carefully avoid minor traffic violations.
3) Don't sneak through yellow lights.
4) Signal well in advance of turning.
5) Maintain proper distance from the vehicle in front of you.
6) Follow all speed control regulations.

Neglecting just one of these precautions, once, can cost a life or a limb.

Does it really matter where you live, in terms of Long Life? Well, **climate has no effect on the rate ofaging**, according to research. In fact, the physical characteristics of a location appear to have less significance than psychological factors such as the promotion of family ties, community involvement, friendships, and the other longevity factors.

For your information, though, I list the States in their order of life expectancy, and the average number of years people live in each State:

STATE	YEARS	STATE	YEARS
1. Hawaii	77.02	27. Indiana	73.84
2. Minnesota	76.15	28. Missouri	73.84
3. Iowa	75.81	29. Arkansas	73.72
4. Utah	75.76	30. New York	73.70
5. North Dakota	75.71	31. Michigan	73.67
6. Nebraska	75.49	32. Oklahoma	73.67
7. Wisconsin	75.35	33. Texas	73.64
8. Kansas	75.31	34. Pennsylvania	73.58
9. Colorado	75.30	35. Ohio	73.49
10. Idaho	75.19	36. Virginia	73.4
11. Washington	75.13	37. Illinois	73.37
12. Connecticut	75.12	38. Maryland	73.32

13. Massachusetts	75.01	39. Tennessee	73.30
14. Oregon	74.99	40. Delaware	73.21
15. New Hampshire	74.98	41. Kentucky	73.06
16. South Dakota	74.97	42. North Carolina	72.96
17. Vermont	74.79	43. West Virginia	72.84
18. Rhode Island	74.76	44. Nevada	72.64
19. Maine	74.59	45. Alabama	72.53
20. California	74.57	46. Alaska	72.24
21. Arizona	74.30	47. Georgia	72.22
22. New Mexico	74.01	48. Mississippi	71.98
23. Florida	74.00	49. South Carolina	71.85
24. New Jersey	74.00	50. Louisiana	71.74
25. Montana	73.93	51. Wash DC	69.20
26. Wyoming	73.85		

Some of the most important factors affecting these figures include health care quality and availability, traffic control, water quality according to mineral content (high selenium content is best), per capita income, air quality (though we have seen no acceptable research drawing a relationship between air quality and years of life, we believe there is a relationship).

Probably the most important consideration in choosing a place to live is how well you like the place, since happiness is such a major factor for Long Life.

The 10 healthiest metropolitan areas based on some of the top longevity factors (fatal traffic accidents, smoking laws, alcohol consumption, pollen count, etc.) are:

Boston, Ma.
Scranton-Wilkes Barre, Pa.
Richmond, Va.
Greensboro, NC.
Pittsburgh, Pa.
Rochester, NY.

Minneapolis-St. Paul, Minn.
Milwaukee, WI.
Honolulu, Ha.
Seattle, WA.

Carl Bourhenne, MA
Gerontologist

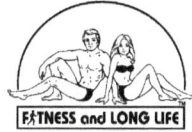

How To Live
The Longest Life Possible

Smoking, Drinking, & Drugs

Don't Smoke!

The relationship between smoking and longevity is so strong that, especially for men in their sixties, smoking is the single most accurate predictor of remaining life expectancy.

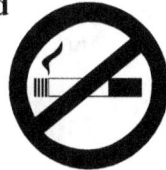

On the average, **cigarette smokers die ten years sooner than otherwise comparable non- smokers**. In addition to causing lung cancer, heart disease, emphysema, and hypertension, cigarette smoking is also a major risk factor for cerebrovascular disease, causing strokes and reducing mental functioning.

It can be said that **all smokers, regardless of age, have a 70% greater probability of experiencing coronary heart disease**. Although the damage from smoking cigarettes can never be reversed, stopping lessens the probability of heart disease.

The body's first reaction to smoking may include sweating, nausea, and even vomiting; but a tolerance to the effects of nicotine is soon developed, and **nicotine is strongly physically addictive**. Unfortunately, the detrimental effects of nicotine remain a danger.

Smoking should be eliminated to avoid or control hypertension. Hypertension can cause damage to all of the body organs, but especially the brain, heart, and kidneys.

Most lung cancers are caused by smoking, and the prognosis for lung cancer is poor. The major cause of the increase in cancer deaths has been the increase of lung cancer. If you stop smoking, your risk of lung cancer is reduced. The risk of developing lung cancer is 10 times as great in an elderly moderate smoker, as that of a no

Both chronic bronchitis and emphysema (collectively known as chronic obstructive lung disease) are usually due to smoking. **No therapy can reverse the lung destruction of emphysema**. Emphysema produces holes in the lung. People with emphysema may be constantly struggling to breathe.

Extreme emphysema is virtually always seen in later years, in long-term heavy smokers. Esophageal carcinoma (Cancer of the esophagus) has been related to smoking, and the prognosis is grave.

Nicotine is a stimulant which causes increases in the blood pressure, heart rate, and the release of epinephrine. Withdrawal symptoms may include headaches, sweating, insomnia, nervousness, and drowsiness.

Contrary to popular belief, **smoking does not relieve stress**. Stress causes an elevation of the acid content in the urine, which in turn flushes away more nicotine than normal urine does. The nicotine addiction then demands a replenishment of the lost nicotine; but the stress level itself remains unaffected. The same tests showed that bicarbonates reduced smoking under stress.

According to the American Cancer Society, a person who smokes two packs of cigarettes per day may expect to live about <u>12 years less</u> than someone who has never smoked.

While those who stop smoking may experience some relief from the effects of emphysema and bronchitis, air sacs destroyed by emphysema can not be recovered, and blocked bronchial airways may never be re-opened.

Substances known as "anaphrodisiacs" are those substances which lessen sexual desire. The most widely used, but least recognized anaphrodisiac is nicotine. **Smoking cigarettes has been shown to reduce sexual motivation and performance**. Nicotine constricts the blood vessels, reducing the body's vasocongestive response to sexual stimulation. Smoking also reduces the levels of testosterone in the blood, further lessening sexual performance.

Smoking is also hazardous to the developing fetus during pregnancy. Smoking cigarettes reduces the amount of oxygen in the bloodstream, and so may slow the growth of the fetus. Thus, babies of mothers who smoked during their pregnancy often weigh less than those of non-smoking mothers.

Research shows that **smoking is associated with skin wrinkling**, probably because nicotine from cigarettes contracts the small blood vessels in the skin, inhibiting circulation.

The Public Health Service's 1975 report, "The Health Consequences of Smoking", states, "Cigarette smoking remains the largest single unnecessary and preventable cause of illness and preventable death". As long ago as 1979 the Secretary of Health, Education, and Welfare and the Surgeon General jointly released a huge report of 1,200 pages entitled Report on Smoking and Health which studied over 30,000 separate, scientific studies. The result was "overwhelming proof" that cigarette smoking causes disease. In it **the HEW Secretary said, "People who smoke are committing slow-motion suicide."**

Way back in 1979 the Surgeon General's report stated that cigarette smoking is responsible for 346,000 deaths each year! Although lung cancer was a relatively rare disease in the year 1900, by 1977 it alone became the killer of 78,000 Americans. Smoking is also responsible for bronchitis, emphysema, cancers of the kidney, pancreas, and bladder; and heart disease.

Arguments have been made in defense of smoking, saying that we tolerate smog, which is also harmful. The fact is that smoke from a typical non-filter cigarette contains about 5 billion particles per milliliter - 50,000 times that of an equal volume of polluted city air.

The strong trend away from non-filter cigarettes toward filtered and low nicotine-low tar cigarettes has not significantly helped. The incidence of lung cancer does drop somewhat, but still remains high. Also, carbon monoxide, along with nicotine, contributes to heart disease; and filtered and low tar-low nicotine cigarettes do not automatically have a low carbon monoxide yield.

It is the tarry substance of cigarette smoke that causes lung cancer. When it is applied to the skin, lungs, and other tissues of rats, mice, and hamsters its compounds produce cancer in the animals. Experiments with dogs showed that when an incision in the trachea of dogs was made in such a way that they were made to smoke seven cigarettes per day for over two years, pre-cancerous changes in the lung tissues developed.

There are other forms of cancer that are directly linked to smoking. Death resulting from cancer of the mouth, larynx, trachea, and esophagus are much higher for smokers than for non-smokers. These types of cancer attack pipe and cigar smokers as readily as cigarette smokers. Leukoplakia, an early form of cancer, develops on the lips, tongue, and mucous membranes of cigar and pipe smokers. As smoking became more widely accepted, cancers of the kidney and pancreas also increased.

Toxic materials derived from smoking are eliminated through the urine. As a result, smokers of a pack of cigarettes per day are twice as likely to die of bladder cancer as are non-smokers.

The difference in heart attacks between smokers and non-smokers is dramatic. Pack-a-day or more cigarette smokers have twice as many heart attacks as non-smokers; and three times as often, the heart attack results in sudden death. Incidences of heart disease increases in direct proportion to the number of cigarettes smoked per day, and the number of years the person has been smoking.

How Does Cigarette Smoke Cause Heart Attacks?
Two of the components of cigarette smoke are carbon monoxide, and nicotine. Carbon monoxide is well known as a colorless, odorless, and very poisonous gas that combines with the hemoglobin in red blood cells, reducing the amount of oxygen that reaches body cells.

Nicotine is one of the toxic substances. It constricts coronary blood vessels and interferes with the nerve signals that regulate the heartbeat. The result is reduced oxygen supply to the heart muscle. This is only one of the problems that nicotine causes. It is suspected of increasing the probability of thrombosis - the formation of blood clots - in the coronary blood vessels, causing heart attack. Other types of strain on the heart caused by nicotine are deteriorated lung functioning, and high blood pressure.

The initial effect of nicotine is a mild stimulation - a lift - but the after effect is a mild depression which stimulates the need for the next cigarette; and so on in a circle.

A 1978 report from the Food and Drug Administration resulted in the labeling of birth control pills with the warning:

"Women who use oral contraceptives should not smoke". The study states that the risk increases with age, and with smoking 15 or more cigarettes per day.

One study showed that women who smoked and used the pill are 22 times more likely to suffer certain kinds of stroke than women who did neither. The 1979 Surgeon General's Report showed that **women who smoke multiply by double the dangers of stillbirths and spontaneous abortions**; and they have babies that are, on the average, a half pound lighter.

The report also stated that **one out of five babies who died could have been saved if the mothers had not been a smokers**.

This same report shows that, after quitting smoking, one's life expectancy improves as the time off of cigarettes increases so that 15 years after quitting, the life expectancy of the ex-smoker is almost the same as that of a non-smoker. This reflects the reductions in the risk of lung cancer and heart attack.

There are many methods of stopping smoking; but, since nicotine is a strong physical addiction, we strongly that anyone wishing to stop smoking get professional help. Some forms of help are very inexpensive; some are low-cost, and some even no-cost. There are such techniques as aversion conditioning, group therapy, emotional role playing, and "cold turkey". There are such groups as the Seventh Day Adventists, who invite anyone who wishes to stop smoking to attend.

In 1970 I, Carl Bourhenne, stopped a 5 (five) pack per day habit in this program, after two years of serious unsuccessful attempts. Religion was not introduced into this wonderful program.

The American Cancer Society, The American Heart Association, and The American Lung Association might develop referral services, clinics or programs. Some hospitals have live-in programs. In considering the cost, remember the several hundred dollars per year the smoker spends on cigarettes.

It is usually only after quitting smoking that the smoker comes to realize the dreadful impact that the smoker has on non-smokers. The acute disturbance of the smoke itself is almost equaled by the ever present tar and nicotine odor and smudge which pervade the path and quarters of the cigarette smoker.

If you're trying to stop smoking: In most cases quitting smoking can best be done with help, such as was mentioned above.

Some brief tips address the real fact that nicotine is a strong physical addiction, as well as mental and emotional:

1) **Certain things stimulate a strong craving for nicotine**, such as the smell of nicotine itself, coffee, alcohol, sweets, and spicy foods, and nicotine in the body. Immediately wash or dry clean the smell of nicotine out of all clothing, curtains and draperies. Flush the nicotine out of your body by eating and drinking nothing but fruit and fruit juices, especially citrus, for 24 hours.

2) **Certain situations stimulate a strong craving for nicotine**, such as the time right after meals, especially when coffee and a cigarette are a habit, when holding a drink, especially at a party, when sitting in front of a cup of coffee, when bored, lonely, or frustrated, when angry, when sad, and at any other times when you are habituated to lighting up. Don't have the coffee after a meal. Instead, get up and go do something. For a while, stop drinking, especially at parties. When emotions are low or high, take appropriate steps to get back on track.

After about a month, it is thought that the smoker's system is past the most difficult stage of quitting. The system is cleaned out, and the person has made a basic (but not complete) adjustment as a non-smoker, so that when someone offers them a cigarette they can truthfully say, "No thanks, I don't smoke."

If the ex-smoker lives long enough, after about fifteen years, the ex-smoker has about the same life expectancy of a non-smoker of the same age, except for the permanent lung damage which may bring on emphysema.

Drinking

Drink alcoholic beverages in moderation, if at all, **don't drive after drinking**. Alcohol is the most widely used intoxicant known to humans. Moderate use can reduce tension and

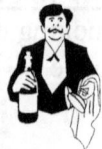

anxiety, and produce a feeling of relaxation and well-being. **It is, in fact, the moderate drinker who lives longer than either the heavy drinker or even the teetotaler.**

More than 50% of all automobile deaths in the United States, and a large number of the injuries involve excessive drinking. Alcohol use is also very often associated with physical illness, mental illness, family conflicts, other social problems, poverty, and crime.

Alcohol is a major factor in the causation of cirrhosis of the liver, which is responsible for over half of all deaths between the ages of 45 and 65. Also, alcohol has been shown to injure the brain and heart.

What is this thing called "alcohol"? What is this most used and abused drug in all of its various popular forms and potencies? Methods of making alcoholic beverages have been known even before recorded history.

There are several classifications of alcoholic beverages:

<u>Beer and Ale</u> contain from 3 to 6 1/2 percent alcohol, and are made from various cereals by brewing.

<u>Table Wines</u> have a natural alcohol content of from 9 to 12 percent alcohol, and are made by fermenting the juice of grapes or other fruits.

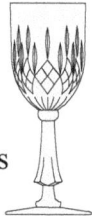

<u>Other Wines</u> such as Ports, Sherries, and Muscatels usually contain 18 to 22 percent alcohol, by the addition of distilled alcohol.

<u>Hard Liquors</u> -- whiskey (bourbon, scotch, etc.), gin, rum, and brandy - contain from 35 to 50 percent alcohol. They are derived by distilling fermented or brewed products to yield these high alcohol liquids.

"**Proof**" on alcoholic beverages indicates the alcohol concentration of a beverage. To convert proof to percent, just divide the proof number in half. For example, 100 proof whiskey is 50 percent alcohol; 80 proof rum is 40 percent alcohol, and so on. Thus, one ounce of 100 proof whiskey contains 1/2 ounce of pure alcohol, etc.

The effect of alcohol on you will be different from other people, in varying degrees.

How a drinking episode affects you will depend on several factors:
   ** Your previous experience with alcohol.
                 ** The strength of the alcoholic beverage.
   ** The rate you consume the beverage.
   ** The rate you absorb the alcohol.
   ** Your body weight (the less you weigh, the less you can handle).
   ** Your own physiological response to alcohol (Some people can drink a lot, and some people can't even take a sip without becoming ill.).
   ** Your motivation for drinking
   ** The impact of your culturalization and socialization to alcohol

Alcohol is carried by the bloodstream to the central nervous system (the brain and spinal cord), and has both physical and psychological effects. It is an anesthetic, a tranquilizer, and a depressant. Because as a tranquilizer it reduces inhibitions - especially in social settings where its effects include increased conversation and activity - it sometimes seems to be a stimulant. The way alcohol induces mood changes though, is to depress the part of the brain involved in sending out instructions to the body. The resulting impairment of motor coordination is the most measurable of the effects of alcohol.

Even moderate amounts of alcohol can increase the heart rate, cause confusion and hallucinations, increase stomach acid and saliva, is a mild diuretic, and dilates blood vessels near the skin giving an illusion of feeling warmer.

Intoxication on a daily basis results in a state of physical dependence and higher tolerance for alcohol. Subsequently, alcohol deprivation results in withdrawal symptoms.

The intensity of the withdrawal symptoms is a good measure of the degree of addiction. Symptoms of withdrawal include seizures, and hallucinations or delirium tremens (DT's).

The "hangover" syndrome is actually a state of mild withdrawal whose severity reflects how much and how long the person drank as well as the person's condition - mentally and physically. Some of the symptoms of a hangover are headache, nausea and vomiting, weakness, nervousness, thought control, and fast heartbeat. **Contrary to popular opinion, there is no cure for a hangover.**

Sadly, none of those odd concoctions, coffee, or vitamins can cure a hangover; but some relief can come from rest, solid food, aspirin, and liquids. Most hangovers have a maximum duration of about 36 hours, and many last only a few hours or less.

Long term heavy drinking results in a high rate of serious illness, both psychological and physical. Mental illness, temporary and permanent can result, as well as stomach and gastrointestinal disorders.

Nutritional disorders are a result of the fact that alcohol is high in calorie, but has no vitamins or essential amino acids, and depresses the appetite. Too much alcohol causes excessive fat deposits and liver tissue damage, resulting in the life-threatening disease known as cirrhosis of the liver.

Other serious effects from excessive alcohol use are various cancers. Especially if the person smokes, cancers of the mouth, pharynx, larynx, and esophagus have been related to heavy drinking.

Heavy drinkers have been shown to have markedly shorter life spans.

From the viewpoint of intoxication, alcohol requires much more intake by volume than most other psychoactive drugs. **Alcohol intoxication occurs after ingestion of between 2 and 4 ounces** - 300 times more than barbiturates, and almost a million times more than LSD. The biggest reason for this is that most of the alcohol ingested does not reach the brain. Alcohol is absorbed into the bloodstream, partly through the lining of the stomach and partly through the small intestine. Then, in the blood, 80 to 90 percent of the alcohol is broken down in the liver and other tissues, with the rest going to the brain.

This last amount, which goes to the brain, is called the "blood alcohol level", and is what determines how much the person's behavior will be affected. If the intake of alcohol is faster than the body can break down and eliminate, the excess alcohol enters the blood stream, raising the "blood alcohol level", and reaches the brain, causing intoxication.

While individuals may vary, most people will notice little or no effect with a concentration of up to .02 percent alcohol in the blood. This amounts to 2 parts of alcohol per 10,000 parts of blood. When the level rises to .03 to .05 percent alcohol, some sensations will ordinarily be noticed, such as a sense of well-being, light-headedness, some relaxation, and some release of personal inhibitions. A person may say or do things they might not ordinarily say or do.

By 0.1 percent blood alcohol concentration the drinker experiences major depression of sensory and motor functions. The drinker will experience difficulty in speaking, and may fumble objects and stagger slightly. At 0.2 percent blood alcohol concentration the drinker will be incapacitated, both mentally and physically. At 0.3 percent the drinker is in a stupor, and at .4 percent, a coma. If the blood alcohol level rises to a level of 0.6 or 0.7 percent, suffocation and death would occur. This is rare, however, because the drinker usually loses consciousness before then, or the stomach becomes irritated and the drinker vomits.

The four major factors to consider in controlling the absorption of alcohol are:

1. The alcohol content of the beverage. The higher the alcohol content, the faster the ingestion of alcohol.
1. Your body weight. The higher your body weight, the more blood you have to dilute the alcohol.
2. The rate of consumption. The faster you drink, the faster you absorb the alcohol in your beverage(s). Chug-a-lugging results in a much faster ingestion than does drinking slowly.
3. The rate of absorption. One of the major factors in rate of absorption is what is in the stomach at the time of drinking. On an empty stomach nothing slows down the absorption process. After a meal, the alcohol absorption process is slower; and, people tend to drink slower. Also, beer slows absorption time slightly, while carbonated sodas used as mixers for the whiskeys tend to accelerate absorption, raising the blood alcohol level faster.

People with certain diseases, such as epilepsy and diabetes should not drink at all. Also, recent illness, and often extreme fatigue may cause an unusual sensitivity to alcohol.

Women who are pregnant should not drink. Even in moderation, drinking can have extremely harmful effects on the unborn baby. "Fetal alcohol syndrome" is a pattern of defects known to be caused by women who are chronic alcoholics. <u>The defects include stunted growth, mental retardation, and malformed faces, hearts, arms, and legs.</u>

Another serious danger regarding alcohol is the interaction of alcohol with drugs. **Any two drugs taken together result in an effect more than the sum of the two drugs, and alcohol is a drug. This includes drinking while using medications.**

In addition to the physical effects of alcohol on people, there are psychological effects. The extent of the effects of a given amount of alcohol depends primarily on the character and personality of the drinker as they interact with both the alcohol and the setting. The psychological effects include both mental impairment, and emotional impairment. The mental impairment which results affects such abilities as motor tasks, reaction time, perception, and the cognitive processes of thinking, reasoning, learning, remembering, and problem solving. The emotional impairment from alcohol consumption includes euphoria, fear, anxiety, tension, and hostility.

With all of the detrimental effects from excessive alcohol consumption, and all of the functional effects of even moderate drinking, more than 100 million Americans above the age of 15 use alcoholic beverages. This includes eight out of ten men, and six out of ten women. The vast majority of those who drink do so without noticeable damage or danger to themselves or others except when they drive after drinking. It is the drinking of alcoholic beverages by about 18 million people who cause injury to others, mostly by driving after drinking. About two-thirds of those are considered alcoholics.

172

Repeated incidences of intoxication which cause problems to oneself or others indicates a drinking problem. People displaying this behavior are called **"problem drinkers"**. Problem drinkers with a physical dependency on alcohol, or who cannot stop drinking once they have started, or who cannot refrain from drinking in inappropriate situations are called **"alcoholics"**.

Some of the indications that a person needs help to deal with an alcohol problem are:
-- Being intoxicated four or more times a year.
-- Needing to drink in order to go to work or school or to a social event.
-- Driving while intoxicated.
-- Being injured and needing medical help as a result of intoxication.
-- Doing something while intoxicated that one feels they would never do while sober.
-- Getting in trouble with the law as a result of drinking.

Efforts to identify the cause of alcoholism have led to research on personality disorders, the effects of culture, liver metabolism, nutritional deficiencies, the central nervous system, hormonal imbalances, and heredity.

Two areas in particular have been identified as initiating factors in the development of alcoholism:

1) Simple learning: A person is lonely, or tense, or otherwise uncomfortable; takes a drink to alleviate it; and becomes more comfortable as a result. This reinforces the behavior, and it eventually becomes an uncontrollable behavioral response to the initiating discomfort.
2) Family: Alcoholism definitely runs in families. This could be due to heredity, or to the family environment, or to both.

There is one alcoholic for every ten drinkers in the United States. Regardless of their pattern of use, they are all seeking the same thing: the intoxicating effects of alcohol. Some only go on occasional binges, and some drink regularly, whether it be all day, or only at night, or only on weekends or holidays. Some cannot stop drinking once they start, until they reach a certain level of intoxication, and some try to maintain an alcoholic euphoria as long as possible.

All types of people become alcoholics, and all alcoholics invariably tend to deny their problem. There are perhaps four male alcoholics to every female alcoholic; but the females are increasing. The highest percentage of alcoholics is no longer among middle-aged men; but is now among men under the age of thirty.

No one knows why yet; but <u>the earlier in life alcoholism develops, the faster it seems to occur</u>. **<u>Teenagers can become alcoholics after only three or four months of alcohol use</u>**; young adults after only two or three years of heavy drinking; and later in life it may occur after six to ten years of heavy, steady drinking.

There is also a significant ethnic association with alcoholism. Because of cultural backgrounds, Americans of Italian (nutritional teachings), Jewish (religious teachings), and Chinese (cultural reasons) heritage have shown low rates of alcoholism.

On the other hand, Americans of Irish and Anglo-Saxon heritage are from cultures which encouraged the use of alcohol to enjoy the intoxicating effects, and have unusually high rates of alcoholism. The longer the families have been exposed to the American culture, however, the more they move toward the national norm.

The treatment of alcoholism calls for encouragement and support from all sides. Ideally, the family, physician, friends, and even employer and work associates are included in discussions of support and treatment. Treatment should include addressing the physical effects of long term drinking, as well as the personality and social factors that may have contributed to the development of alcoholism.

The first emphasis in treatment should be full acceptance of the problem drinker as an ill person needing long term treatment on an outpatient basis.

In addition to the physician, professional treatment is usually necessary. The well-known organization, **Alcoholics Anonymous (AA)** may still be the leading source of such treatment. Their services are free, and are based on mutual support and understanding of the special problems of alcoholism through personal experience. This organization is nation-wide.

In addition, **support for the spouses of alcoholics is provided by the organization Al-Anon**; and at the organization.

Alateen the teen-age children of alcoholics are able to meet to help one another.

Physicians sometimes use Antabuse (disulfiram). This is used in a tablet form, and is taken daily. It produces a toxic reaction if any alcohol is consumed, causing severe nausea. It can help the alcoholic remain sober while receiving other needed treatment, such as individual and group psychotherapy, vocational counseling, social work services, and other approaches used in combination with AA and Antabuse.

It is the "light drinker" (no more than 1 drink, 1 glass of wine, or 1 beer per day) who tends to live longer than either the abstainer, or those who drink more. **If you are a "light drinker" (no more than 1 drink, 1 glass of wine, or 1 beer per day), you can expect to live two to ten years longer, and be healthier than those who drink more**; all other considerations being equal.

If you are a "moderate drinker" of 2, 3, or 4 drinks in the course of a day, you are losing ground daily in the maintenance of your health; and **you are likely to live at least two to six years less than if you were a "light drinker"**. At this stage of the game, you could probably cut down on your own. If you have difficulty in doing so, you should get help, immediately.

Those who drink to excess, however, have markedly shorter life spans. This is due in part to the development of liver disease, which in turn allows the development of a number of other health problems. If you are a "heavy drinker" (more than 4 drinks per day), you may have already frankly considered yourself an alcoholic. If not, you should immediately consult a helpful organization that will support you in arriving at an accurate assessment of your drinking problem. And **as a "heavy drinker" you definitely do have a drinking problem, which will most likely kill you at least 5 to 15 years early**.

DRUGS

Hard drugs are clearly deadly, and are a downhill path to physical, mental, and emotional destruction. So-called "soft" drugs are also dangerous - especially since they are progressive and/or harmful to the mind and body; especially the nervous system.

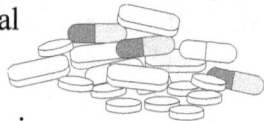

"Crack" cocaine ("rocks") are perhaps the most addictive, and for most people, one puff can result in lifetime addiction.

The most harmful of all the drugs might be "Angel Dust", or PCP, since every puff causes permanent brain damage.

Research on marijuana is exposing uses of a true medicinal nature for the treatment of glaucoma, arthritis, and several other ailments. It may be prescribed by a doctor in certain states for these uses, as well as for the relief of the nausea caused by chemotherapy.

Carl Bourhenne, MA
Gerontologist

Carl Bourhenne's

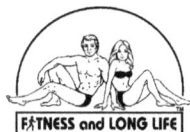

FITNESS and LONG LIFE

How To Live
The Longest Life Possible

Skin Care and Rejuvenation

One of the most obvious factors influencing the way that we attract or do not attract each other - and especially the opposite sex - is the appearance of our skin. Recent studies have provided a new and clearer understanding or our skin, and of what makes it healthy, youthful, and attractive, or wrinkled, sagging, spotted, and aged looking.

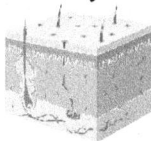

The results of perhaps the most significant research is best summarized by presenting the findings of Dr. Irvin Blank of Harvard Medical School. Dr. Blank proved that dry skin is not necessarily the result of a loss of natural oils. This recent discovery lead the way into an entirely new approach to skin care by major cosmetic manufacturers.

Dr. Blank's research showed that the presence of water in the skin is primarily responsible for keeping skin moist and flexible. He allowed a piece of a callous to lose its water while retaining its natural oils, and it became hard and brittle. He then soaked it in oils used in the most expensive skin care products, but it did not soften. In fact, in one study he left it immersed for seventeen years, and till it remained hard and dehydrated. But, when he immersed the dried piece of callous in water, it quickly softened and became flexible.

Dr. Blank also removed the natural oils from a skin sampling, but caused it to retain its water. The skin sampling retained its softness and flexibility, thus showing the greater importance of water over natural oils in maintaining skin softness. As a result of this research, many cosmetic manufacturers immediately raced to put a new product on the market known as "moisturizers".

As a matter of fact, **the best skin moisturizer is plain mineral water in the form of steam, or spray**.

However, oils can and do soften the outer layer of hardened skin somewhat; but even better, they tend to retain the natural oils inside the skin by sealing them in from dehydration caused by the sun, the wind, and, perhaps the sea spray.

Skin care, and skin rejuvenation are both accomplished by similar techniques. When we utilize the methods of caring for our skin but intensify them, we perform the procedures for rejuvenating damaged skin.

There are two kinds of methods for skin care, and these methods are both strict requirements for keeping, or for regaining and maintaining healthy, youthful, attractive skin:
1) Care from the outside
2) Provision from the inside

1) Care from the outside: The skin must be kept moist and pliable so that it does not dry and crack, causing wrinkles. This is best done by using good quality moisturizers. Also, when in the sun, always use a sunscreen to avoid burning and drying of the skin. The weather, more than any other factor in the normal

environment, has the most damaging effect on the skin.

2) <u>Provision from the inside:</u> The skin must receive nutrients to maintain, rebuild, and reproduce healthy skin cells. Vitamins A, E, C, and poly-unsaturated fats are essential for the body to maintain its skin in a healthy, youthful, and attractive, condition.

The effects of stress are especially harmful to the skin, because stress depletes our system of many nutrients - particularly of Vitamin C, which is so necessary to maintain the health of collagen. Collagen is the material which binds the skin cells together. When the collagen in our skin becomes unhealthy it becomes brittle, then when the skin bends it cracks, causing wrinkles.

The skin is actually an organ - the largest and most visible organ in the body. The skin cells reproduce themselves as fast and as often as any other type of cell in the body if cared for, and if provided with the materials needed to repair and reproduce themselves.

The main considerations for skin care and rejuvenation:

1) Since weather has the most devastating effect on the skin, keep a sun block and a moisturizer on the skin of the face, neck, backs of the hands, and all other exposed skin areas when outdoors. Ever notice how some people with wrinkled faces, necks, and hands sometimes have the body of a youngster? These are excellent examples of how the weather ages the exposed skin areas.

2) Whenever the face feels dry, or the facial skin feels tight, moisturize immediately.

3) Provide your skin daily with the nutrients it must have to repair and replace itself, especially vitamins A, E, C, and poly-unsaturated fats; and drink plenty of water.

4) Perform at least 15 minutes of strenuous exercise - not related to work of any kind - for circulation, so that the nutrients will be delivered to the skin, especially in the upper parts of the body such as the face and neck.

5) Avoid junk foods - especially sugar, but also all condensed carbohydrates. They clog the circulatory system and prevent the delivery of oxygen and nutrients to the various skin area.

6) As much as possible, avoid, or immediately relieve stress. After any stressful experience, take some vitamins C, and E. Stress drains the body of them, and the body does not store them.

8) Avoid habitual extremes of facial expression, which can develop into wrinkles. Keep a relaxed and pleasant face to keep it smooth and wrinkle free.

9) As much as possible keep your environment humid to keep your skin moist. A vaporizer or humidifier can be used to keep the air moist.

10) If you lie in the sun, always use a good quality sunscreen as described below. Don't lie in direct sunlight between the hours of 10:00 A.M. and 3:00 P.M., and when you lie in the sun use a sunscreen of at least 15 SPF (This means that 15 hours with SPF 15 = 1 hour without a sunscreen.).

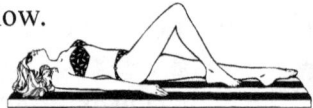

Direct Sunlight Ages The Skin Very Rapidly, And Causes Skin Cancer.

This is the story on the sun's rays:

UV-A: Deep penetrating rays. Excess can cause malignant melanoma, the most deadly form of skin cancer.

UV-B: Burns and damages the surface layers of the kin, and causes such skin cancers as basal cell carcinoma, etc.

UV-C is blocked by the earth's ozone layer.

Sun Lamps such as those used in tanning salons use the longer UV-A rays, which can cause the most dangerous type of skin cancer, malignant melanoma. They don't use the shorter UV-B rays because those are the rays that burn the surface of the skin, causing "sunburn".

If you must be in the sun, protect yourself by using a good quality waterproof sunscreen of SPF (Sun Protection Factor) of 15 or greater, that contains benzophenones and cinnamates, which absorb both UVA and UVB light.

PABA absorbs only UVB rays, so it prevents "sunburn" of the surface of the skin, but since it does not block UV-A rays, it does not prevent malignant melanoma, the most dangerous form of skin cancer.

The sunscreen should be applied to all parts of the body that are to be exposed, prior to exposure. **The most important thing to remember about using sunscreens is to use them frequently and generously.**

SPF-15 means that 15 hours in the sun with the sunscreen is equal to 1 hour in the sun without it. SPF lotions of greater than 15 do not appear to provide significantly greater protection than does SPF-15

As a final motivating inducement to encourage a plentiful provision of vitamins A, E, and C, I offer an interesting note which we encountered in our research: Vitamins A, E, and C can help deter for some people what is known as "liver spots", those dark blotches seen on the skin of some older people. These spots are also known by the "beautiful people" as the lovely-sounding, but off-putting name of "fleur-de-cimetiere" (flower of the cemetery), which seems to suggest that they could be a precursor of death itself.

Some people have surprisingly youthful skin, even at advanced ages. We have already explained the major reasons.

Our research clearly shows that, aside from hereditary factors - which are very relevant indeed - the youthfulness and attractiveness of your skin is quite controllable by adherence to the directions that provided here.

NEW SKIN

There are two effective methods for replacing a very wrinkled and spotted face with a new, smooth, youthful face:
1 . Chemical peeling
2 . Dermabrasion

There are many successful histories from each method, but some unsuccessful results were also noted - mainly as a result of allergic reaction, or of extremely sensitive skin.

Chemical peeling is more risky, as severe allergic reactions have resulted in permanent facial damage to a few people. Many Board Certified Plastic Surgeons (the only practitioners one should go to for this treatment) stay away from Chemical Peeling, except for spot applications on the upper lip, or where Dermabrasion causes too much bleeding. In Southern areas, where the sun has developed too leathery a skin for Dermabrasion to be effective, Chemical Peeling is more common.

Chemical Peeling is performed by applying a phenol solution to the face, to effect a controlled chemical burning of the skin. This results in a really awful full-face scab, which comes loose in about a week. The result is a truly new and youthful face. Don't plan on tanning afterward however, since a peeled skin is essentially a controlled burn scar, and scars don't tan. That is one of the costs of this procedure: you can't tan your face once you've done it.

The cost ranges from $1,200 to $2,500 for a full face job; and $100 or so for spot applications.

The newer procedures for Chemical Peeling use a gradual process in which the skin layers are removed little by little over a period of months. The procedure is once a week for three weeks, then biweekly for six weeks, then once every third week until the desired result is achieved.

2. Dermabrasion is more easily controlled. The epidermis is deadened using a local anesthetic, and then frozen with a refrigerant spray that further reduces pain, inhibits bleeding, and firms up the skin. This process involves bleeding. The Plastic Surgeon (Board Certified in COSMETIC Surgery, please) then uses a tiny rotating wire brush to scrape off the outer layer of skin. Expect to devote a full morning to this procedure, and one to two weeks for healing. A new epidermis will grow, and you will tan naturally afterward. The cost is $2,000 to $3,500; and the results can be truly amazing.

Plastic Surgery

Now that the entire approach to Plastic Surgery is a commonly accepted option for everyone, to improve upon their attractiveness and regain a youthful appearance, more and more women and men from all walks of life are choosing, and using that option. No longer is cosmetic surgery a tool only for those in show business, fashion, or the beauty industry. Men and women, middle class as well as the rich, office worker, public relations worker; all are taking advantage of the perfected skills of the board certified plastic surgeon.

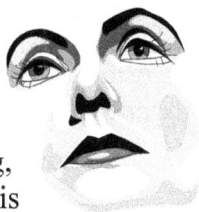

Before going any further I want to point out, and emphasize the vital importance of **seeing only a Board Certified Plastic Surgeon, Experienced With Cosmetic Surgery.** Then, get some references from that surgeon, or people who had the same work done that you are considering; then, speak with each of those references. They are usually eager to share their experience. If you get any hesitation from the plastic surgeon on proving **board certification in Cosmetic surgery**, or providing references, make fast tracks out of there!

The problem here is that any medical doctor is legally licensed to perform plastic surgery; but might have neither the training nor the experience.

The number of people who have been permanently disfigured by the well-meaning, but untrained physician is still mounting. To be Board Certified, the plastic surgeon must undergo several additional years of specialized education and training. Use only him or her.

There are four major types of plastic surgery:
1) Catastrophic surgery (to correct the results of burns and accidents).
2) The correction of congenital anomalies (cleft lips, nose and ear deformities, etc.)
3) Cancer surgery and reconstruction (as related to the face, neck, and breasts).
4) Cosmetic surgery (for improvement of the appearance).

The fourth, Cosmetic Surgery, actually can and usually does improve the quality and enjoyment of one's life, under the right conditions. Look for improvement though, never for miracles.

Your plastic surgeon must be certified by The American Board Of Plastic Surgery, and trained in Cosmetic Surgery, (Not just reconstructive surgery).

You can call your regional Medical Association, and ask them what specialties the surgeon you are considering is board certified for. You might also call your regional "Society of Plastic Surgery".

Look twice at the big advertiser of Plastic Surgery, since their high advertising costs can put additional pressure on them, which may cause them to give less personal attention to the individual patient.

And beware of the surgeon who wants you to have work done on the first day that you see him or her. There's no rush. You want to check him or her, and his or her references. It's your face.

Beware also of the surgeon who tells you he has a new, secret technique. Leave his office, but fast! **It is illegal to have a medical secret.** Besides, you hardly want to be a guinea pig for someone's "bright idea".

What I'm trying to say, of course, is - Don't become one of the many plastic surgery "butcher stories" that result from incompetent practitioners.

But don't be turned off by fear, either. Just make sure the surgeon you engage is a Board Certified Plastic Surgeon, in Cosmetic surgery. If you have the slightest doubt, keep looking!

The valid needs of the woman who thinks her husband's eyes may be roving toward younger girls, and the executive who's younger looking juniors are starting to show real talent can both be re-enforced by cosmetic surgery and the accompanying personal changes in lifestyle, wardrobe, grooming, and make-up.

Very often, in fact, lifestyle changes alone, such as new eating and drinking habits, a vigorous exercise program, wardrobe and grooming improvements, and other lifestyle improvements can make an even greater impact on one's appearance than was ever hoped with cosmetic surgery. In fact, we believe that anyone considering cosmetic surgery might first make the lifestyle changes which will support the new image, especially if weight loss is called for. Of course, no cosmetic surgery is designed as a substitute for dieting. If you are overweight, a good plastic surgeon should have you lose your excess weight before surgery.

There is a new procedure for removing deep facial wrinkles, by laser. The old way, using the chemical phenol, was extremely painful, and required weeks of painful recovery. The new method, though, uses a carbon dioxide laser under local anesthetic, and is entirely painless. The old, wrinkled skin just falls away, replaced by new, youthful looking skin.

As the popularity of cosmetic surgery has increased and broadened, so has its technology. Cosmetic surgery now deals not only with the face, but also includes what is artistically called "body sculpting". Perhaps the most popular form of "body sculpting" is breast augmentation. The surgeon makes an incision under the breast, lifts the entire gland away form the chest wall, and inserts a chemically inert sac filled with one of several jelly-like fluids.

Never allow injections of free-flowing substances into your body. It often migrates throughout the body, causing any of a number of serious problems. This is a process you, yourself, could learn to do in about fifteen minutes, and the results are very often disastrous.

Other successful uses of "body sculpting" by cosmetic surgery produced by our research are: The tightening of flabby skin after weight loss or pregnancy, elimination of stretch marks, the tightening of stomach muscles to flatten the tummy, and the tightening of other areas of body skin after weight loss - such as the underarms, thighs, buttocks, and breasts.

The most popular forms of Plastic Surgery are described in the following sections:

Sagging Eyes (Blepharoplasty): This operation of removing the bags under the eyes and tightening up the eyelids is generally considered a relatively permanent procedure. Very few people require it more than once, as the results are quite lasting. The loose skin is simply slit, the excess skin removed, and the skin sewn up again, hiding the faint scars in the natural crease of the eye. You can return to work in a few days, wear dark glasses for a couple of weeks until the incisions heal, and look a little "wide-eyed" until the scar areas relax (a few months). This procedure requires only a couple of hours under a local anesthetic; and the operation is not disabling. The cost is $2,000 to $6,000.

Forehead Lift: The heavily wrinkled, or "corrugated" forehead can be alleviated. The surgeon slices the scalp well up in the hair and from ear to ear, trims off the excess skin, pulls up the remaining skin and smoothes it out, like smoothing out a sheet. Care must be taken by the surgeon not to try for too dramatic a result by pulling too hard, or permanently raised eyebrows and a slightly receding hairline can result. This procedure works quite well for both men and women, and very often a few hair plugs are transplanted to return the widow's peak to normal. The cost is $2,000 to $6,000.

Small Veins In The Legs - not the large varicose veins, but the smaller, dark ones - can be eliminated by a vascular surgeon. A procedure called "sclerosing injection for superficial venules of the lower extremities" is now being used. A solution is injected into the small, bluish veins in the legs, and they go away. It is important to have this done only by a vascular surgeon experienced in this particular technique, since my research did pick up some problems. In competent hands however, the technique is excellent. It is most commonly done in Los Angeles.

Nose Job (Rhinoplasty): The nose job is now quite common, and is widely accepted as a way of changing the shape of the nose. The procedure is as varied as the type of job being done, so I'll include no technical detail here. It is probably the most easily and dependably successful form of cosmetic surgery, all things considered. The cost is $2,000 to $5,000.

Breast Reduction: It is more complicated, and thus more costly to reduce the size of the breast than it is to enlarge them. There are many methods and many options, so I won't include details here. Your surgeon will explain the options that are available to you, personally. The cost will be $3,500 to $10,000.

Tummy Tuck (Abdominal lipectomy): The Tummy Tuck can include a tightening of both the skin and the abdominal muscles. The cost: $2,000 to $5,000.

Otoplasty: Otoplasty is pinning back prominent ears. Cost $750 to $3,000.

For the above procedures, the cost shown all reflect only the surgeon's fee, and do not include hospital expenses. Most all of these procedures, though, can be performed as an outpatient service. Practically no medical insurance plans cover elective surgery. If the surgeon uses the ambulatory surgical unit of a hospital, the facilities fee will be $600 to $2,000, but if the surgeon operates in his own office, the fee should be more like $300 to $900. If you wish to be put to

190

sleep during the procedure, the fee for the anesthesiologist will run about 20% of the amount of the surgeon's fee.

Cosmetic surgery is recognized by the Internal Revenue Service as a legitimate medical expense deduction.

Some people still tend to believe that cosmetic surgeons can perform miracles. They cannot change personalities, make marriages happy, or get anyone a better job. The changes they make should make you look more rested, relaxed, healthier, younger, and more attractive, but the effect on one's happiness is up to the individual. It is, however, rather common for one of the effects of cosmetic surgery to be a change in self-image and thus, general outlook - which can dramatically change one's life enjoyment. The amount of change is usually in direct proportion to the improvement in lifestyle.

Carl Bourhenne, MA
Gerontologist

Carl Bourhenne's

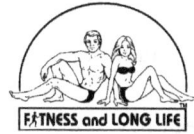

How To Live
The Longest Life Possible

Hair Care

Want to know the Truth about Minoxidil? (Rogaine is one of the brand names). This relatively new treatment acts in various ways; but generally, results are as follows: On those bald or balding pates, slight hair growth was seen in 60% of the subjects tested, in the form of "vellus hair", more commonly known as "peach fuzz". This slight growth was observed for 12 to 14 months, after which time the Minoxidil had no further effect. The slight increased growth then disappeared and treatment was discontinued. Most noticeable results of this treatment were seen when Minoxidil was used with retinoic acid (Retin-A).

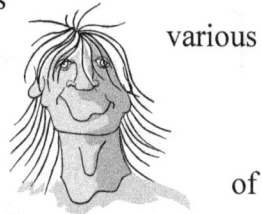

There is, though, a newer and perhaps more promising treatment than minoxidil for the balding or thinning head: The active agent is zomexin, and is derived from the lining of the stomachs of pigs. Hair loss was stopped in 90% of the subjects tested in an informal study, and 65% of the subjects grew vellus hair.

Perhaps the most disturbing thing about losing hair or going bald is the effect that it might have on one's love life, especially as a single person. The loss of love and sex appeal is very threatening. Most people realize that persons of the opposite sex who prefer "the balding look" are in the minority.

The first response to an awareness of balding is styling the hair to cover the balding areas. Subsequent responses include hair and scalp massage, and the consideration of various types of hair rejuvenation and hair replacement methods. Fortunately there are such good hair replacements available today that no one, not close friends, or lovers, or even mothers can detect them even when touched and pulled, or tugged on moderately hard. This, of course, is the most desirable requisite of any hair replacement method.

In order to know what to do for the hair, it is helpful to know what makes hair grow. The scalp contains tens of thousands of hair follicles, and each produces one hair. Hair follicles are shaped like a bulb with a small tube extending from it. They are nourished by papillae; cone-shaped elevations at the base of the hair follicle. The follicles produce cells in the bulb area. When the bulb is filled and cell division continues, the cells push their way out the tube portion of the follicle.

While enroot to the scalp surface these cells stop dividing, and a substance called keratin is produced (keratin is also found in the nails). Then the hair is forced to the scalp surface by the continuing cell production in the bulb area of the follicle.

This is the active cycle of hair growth, which continues for about five years in a healthy follicle. Then the active cycle subsides, and the follicle adopts a resting stage. This resting stage lasts about three months, and then the follicle resumes cell production. A new shaft then pushes the old shaft out, and it is shed. The average person sheds 80 to 120 hairs each day, in this manner.

Many things can traumatize an excessive number of follicles into the resting stage, such as high temperature, a serious illness, some medicines, poisons, and some anesthetics. Hair loss may show up two to three months later.

Some women experience hair loss due to a decrease in estrogen after giving birth, or after starting or stopping use of birth control pills.

Hair loss due to any of these reasons is temporary, and when the body returns to normal, so does hair growth. New hair again appears after a few months.

All Serious scalp problems should be treated by a dermatologist.

Although dandruff does not cause hair loss, it can readily lead to it. Certain physical disturbances of the scalp can cause hair loss. Some examples are habitual wearing of tight headgear, tight curlers, tight hair-do's, teasing the hair, excessive use of chemicals (dyes, permanents, straighteners, bleaches, and sprays), and an over or under active thyroid.

The most common cause of baldness in men is "Male Pattern Baldness". It is attributed to heredity. All normal men see some recession of the hair line by the age of 20. Eunuchs, however, will never lose their hair. In fact, in countries where castration has been used, some significant facts are noted: When castration occurs before puberty, the hairline of a young boy is maintained throughout life, even if he has a long family history of male pattern baldness. And when a balding man - even a man balding due to male pattern baldness - is castrated, all hair loss stops. These results are due to the absence of the male hormone testosterone, which is manufactured in the testes.

It might seem to follow that mental attitudes stressing excessive virility, such as, "men don't cry", extreme independence, high regimentation, and insufficient sexual activity might cause higher levels of testosterone to be present in the system to act on the hair follicles, contributing to hair loss.

Carl Bourhenne, MA
Gerontologist

Carl Bourhenne's

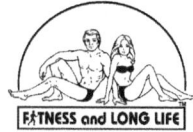

FITNESS and LONG LIFE

How To Live
The Longest Life Possible

Your Inherited Genes

Our beautiful bodies and our intelligent brains are entirely the product of the genes which we inherited from our parents. Each one of our genes, and the combinations of our genes are crucial to the way that we look and function. Perhaps no single fact shows this more dramatically than the small, yet so notable gene differences between man and the chimpanzee: Anthropologists tell us that we are evolutionary descendants of the chimpanzee. These creatures seem so very different from us, and yet our genes are 98.2 percent identical to the chimpanzee! So each one of our genes, and our gene combinations are vital to our make-up and our health.

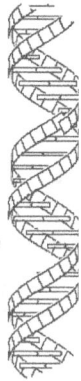

In additional to determining our make-up, our genes also determine how healthy we will be, and how long we can live. As I mentioned in the OVERVIEW, the research of Richard G. Cutler of the National Institute on Aging, National Institutes of Health has shown that our genes presently limit human lifespan to an absolute maximum of about 120 years.

197

I mentioned that Cutler's studies of the evolution of human genes shows that, although the lifespan of our evolving species was growing rapidly, it leveled off about 100,000 years ago at about 120 years, and has remained there ever since. Once the mapping of the human genome is completed, Genetic Engineering may extend our youthful health and lifespan by...who knows how much? And, as I also pointed out in the OVERVIEW, diseases and handicaps of all kinds may slide into history, just as penicillin and other "miraculous" advancements have put so many infirmities into our history. Once the mapping of the human genome is completed, Genetic Engineering may allow us to cure and prevent every illness known to man, and even re-grow lost body parts. And since our genes control our lifespan, who knows how much we could extend the length of our lives?

In order to best use the information available to us, such as the information in **How To Live The Longest Life Possible**, we must each look at our own genes as closely as possible and make special provisions for the weaknesses that we each may have inherited.

Each of us must pay special attention to our genetic background in order to provide for our own special needs for preventive medicine, special nutrition, and the other lifestyle factors that promote health and long life.

We can each adopt two strategies to assess our own genes: We can look at our family history ourselves and observe the health and longevity factors of our relatives and predecessors, and we can hire the services of a geneticist to do a more in-depth study.

The results could be the avoidance of minor and major illnesses, and the maximization of our own potential lifespan.

After assessing our genes we can contact the appropriate organizations for guidance in maximizing our health and long life. For example, if we have a family history of heart trouble, we can contact the American Heart Association for guidance. If there is a family history of a particular type of cancer, we contact one of the major cancer research organizations such as the American Cancer Society, and so on.

There is a new area of medicine called **"Darwinian Medicine"**, which examines the traits developed during the long line of the evolution of man. One of the goals is to look at our inherited traits with the view toward compensating for those traits which are no longer useful and might be harmful, and enhancing those traits which are indeed beneficial.

It is important to note that we do not necessarily inherit any particular characteristic of either of our parents. Our gene pool is affected by previous generations as well as by our own parents. In fact, generally speaking, we stand only about a 25 percent chance of displaying any one particular characteristic of either of our parents. Whether or not we display a particular parental characteristic is the result of a combination of "dominant" and "recessive" genes which we inherited from both of them for that characteristic.

The information in "**How To Live The Longest Life Possible**" is generally for everyone. Adjustments may be made in the use of the information, based on your personal genetic background, **but only after consulting your physician.**

Carl Bourhenne, MA
Gerontologist

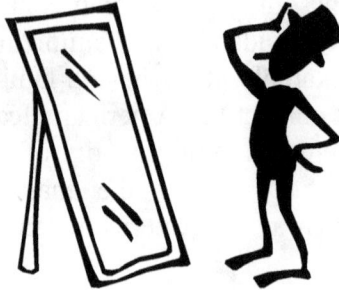

THE ONE IN THE GLASS

When You Get What You Want In Your Struggle For Self
    And The World Lets You Rule For A Day,
Then Go To The Mirror And Look At Yourself,
    And See What The Mirror Has To Say.

For It Isn't Your Mother, Or Father, Or Lover
    Whose Judgment Upon You Must Pass.
The Person Whose Verdict Counts Most In Your Life
    Is The One Looking Back From The Glass.

That's The Person To Please, Never Mind All The Rest.
    That One's With You Clear To The End.
You've Passed Your Most Dangerous, Difficult Test
    If The One In The Glass Is Your Friend.

You May Be Like Jack Horner And Chisel A Plum,
    And Think You're A Wonderful Spy.
But The One In The Glass Says You're Only A Bum,
    If You Can't Look 'Em Straight In The Eye.

You Can Fool The World On The Pathway Of Years,
    And Get Pats On The Back As You Pass.
But Your Final Reward Will Be Heartaches And Tears,
    If You've Cheated The One In The Glass.

Carl Bourhenne, MA
Gerontologist

www.ingramcontent.com/pod-product-compliance
Lightning Source LLC
Chambersburg PA
CBHW061735270326
41928CB00011B/2246